The Reluctant Carer

The Reluctant Carer

Dispatches from the Edge of Life

PICADOR

First published 2022 by Picador
an imprint of Pan Macmillan
The Smithson, 6 Briset Street, London ECIM 5NR
EU representative: Macmillan Publishers Ireland Limited, 1st Floor,
The Liffey Trust Centre, 117–126 Sheriff Street Upper
Dublin 1 D01 YC43
Associated companies throughout the world
www.panmacmillan.com

ISBN 978-1-5290-2935-2

1 3 5 7 9 8 6 4 2

A CIP catalogue record for this book is available from the British Library.

Typeset by Palimpsest Book Production Ltd, Falkirk, Stirlingshire
Printed and bound by CPI Group (UK) Ltd, Croydon, CRO 4YY

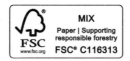

Visit **www.picador.com** to read more about all our books
and to buy them. You will also find features, author interviews and
news of any author events, and you can sign up for e-newsletters
so that you're always first to hear about our new releases.

The pleasure of being necessary to my parents was profound.
I was not like the children in folktales: burdensome mouths
to feed, nuisances to be corrected, problems so severe that
they were abandoned to the forest. I had a status.

TONI MORRISON, *THE NEW YORKER*

You're on earth, there's no cure for that!
SAMUEL BECKETT, *ENDGAME*

Up the Hill Backwards

I forget who rang, but I remember the call.

No one was certain which my of my father's ailments had jumped the queue, but there were plenty of contenders. Heart, kidneys, or those beleaguered, low-tar lungs? The smart money would be on something respiratory, but we were deep in extra time already. Any smart money fled long ago.

These calls come, sooner or later. Wherever you are in your 'journey', as they say. The collapse of a loved one, or someone you are supposed to love, will abduct you into another reality.

The question is how readily we sign up for the ride.

As my mother or my sister or my brother outlined the details of the Old Man's latest hospital admission, I paced the upstairs of my home. This was where we took important calls because the signal was clear.

'Let me figure out what to do,' I said. Then I hung up the phone.

The knot in my stomach was already forming the opinion that I didn't want to go back. Back to the house where my parents lived and I was mostly raised, now seventy miles from my own.

I had left them just the day before. Dad was eighty-six then. Mum, eighty-eight, fitter than my father, but fragile all the same. There was always something that needed doing and it was good just to be around. Even if all each visit did was make it easier to leave again, it was better than nothing. Besides, I liked being there. Up to a point. It still resembled childhood, somehow. Much older actors, but essentially the same play. And at that point still one I could walk out of.

They were in their forties when they had me, twelve years after my sister and nine since my brother. On holidays, the other kids sometimes thought my parents were my grandparents. This worried me, but I was worried already. Mentally preparing for their deaths and all deaths since I realized mortality was the price of being around. I was seven years old, in the same room where I am writing this now, reading a storybook about birds, when it hit me. One bird died and the other birds could neither revive it nor accept its passing. I ran downstairs in a panic and asked my mother if we would both die.

'Yes,' she told me. 'But not for a very long time.'

Right on both counts.

It is the answered prayers that we have to watch out for, and their long lives were mine.

Dad spent four decades in the merchant navy and I watched his fettle turn for the worse in recent years as slowly and surely as one of his ships. The nature of his work meant I didn't see much of him growing up. By the time he retired I had left home. Yet in each of these more frequent crises, by some eerie symmetry, I was with him. As if we had been sailing back towards each other all along. Or rather he lay in wait, floating. Just beneath the surface . . . like a mine.

This call was different. I could sense it, and I knew because I didn't want to know. Despite decades of planning, fretting and elaborate internal bargaining, I felt no more qualified to take this on board at forty-seven than at seven.

I went downstairs to tell my wife.

'Dad's in hospital again. I don't know what difference it makes if I'm there. I just got back. Maybe I can wait and see what happens . . .'

Having crossed the Atlantic countless times to nurse her mother through a quarter-century of cancer, she turned from her cooking and said simply –

'Go.'

My brother was nearby and picked me up. Ninety minutes later we arrived.

We moved into this house in 1976, that fabled summer of parched verges and punk rock. I daresay the five tall, smooth-tiled steps up to the front door seemed, like cigarettes and unprotected sex, to be a good idea at the time.

They have been cracked by the subsequent seasons, acquired a grab rail and attain, in rain or winter, the kind of dreadful status in the minds of those who dwell atop them as K2 and the Eiger hold for mountaineers.

No one old or sober has yet fallen all the way down them, but as I hauled my bag indoors that day I was falling up them, in a sense. Out of one life and into another. A mile away, in hospital, Dad was on the margins, but it was my world that was really changing. Having pitched his tent at death's door long before it opened, like an anxious early drinker, or a shopper waiting on the sale, he was braced for what was coming. I was in for a surprise.

*

In those nine months Dad managed a partial rebound which allowed him and his rolling buffet of comorbidities home, and, shortly after, I abandoned mine. My marriage, like my father, was less stable than it seemed and my wife and I are in the foothills of divorce. Irreversibly so.

In what turned out to be a synchronous skip fire of a season, my work evaporated at the same time as one grand self-employed gamble went gratuitously wrong, and it will take years to get back to that point again, if I ever do. So my somehow-recovering father was tended to by a quietly collapsing version of his son. Ready at your bedside, bedraggled with errors, out of money, as well as love, luck and lodging. As the year trudged on I found myself subtly and circumstantially absorbed into my parents' house and rituals, the gaps between what they can, can't and shouldn't do.

Gradually, I become a carer. My siblings have kids and karma of their own. They work. I have no children, job, money or anyone else to worry about now. This is how I came to be back in the town and the bedroom I left in the late eighties, caring for people in their late eighties. Sure, I care. But I am also captive. And care sounds better than failure. All I really have is nowhere else to go.

'Don't care was made to care!' my mother used to say to me, an admonishment fashioned from an old rhyme. And so it came to pass.

Up the Hill Backwards

Don't care didn't care,
Don't care was wild:
Don't care stole plum and pear
Like any beggar's child.
Don't care was made to care,
Don't care was hung:
Don't care was put in a pot
And boiled till he was done.

PART ONE

Everybody Hurts

1 November 2017

People ask me what I want: friends, lawyers, bartenders. I have no idea. Some days a time machine, others a gun. Most mornings I don't even ask myself. The first question in this house is always, 'Did we make it through the night?'

Once a rustle, a cough or a groan confirms our group survival then the big issue dissolves into the everyday details and desires of any other household – can I make it to the bathroom before you?

Dad's ablutions unfold at a subglacial rate which means I do not want to miss my slot before he gets in there and stays put for the duration of the average movie. That he gets to the bathroom at all is a wonderful thing. It wasn't always so and is by no means certain. But I still don't want to get stuck behind him. If nothing else, being back at home has proven a radical affirmation that you can be grateful and selfish at the same time.

Joint first on the everyday wish list is that my mother – eighty-nine now, and presently felled by shingles – doesn't make it downstairs before me and start doing things for herself when she is this unwell. She has a determination which, through infirmity, borders on self-destruction, and will, like some crazed Olympian, attempt everything she can unless someone intervenes.

Despite the considerable edge in years and mobility, my winning this slow-paced race is not a given. I don't want to get up and face things, and I won't until I hear one of them stirring. Only then will I burst forth belatedly and either get into the bathroom first (which annoys Dad) or intercept Mum (which startles and confuses her). I had hoped the adolescent stasis of lying in bed and wrangling negative outcomes would have fallen away in middle age, but not yet. If anything, it's back with a vengeance, like me, in the same bed where it began. A truly wise person once told me that people don't change, they just become more of who they are. I see little in this house to refute that.

Once we are up and running (there is no running), I conduct a series of interviews with the key players and get a sense of what we might do today. The first conversation of the day is always about sleep. 'How did you sleep?' 'Did you sleep OK?' 'How are you?' Out of this comes a kind of competitive insomnia. 'Oh, it was awful.' 'Up all night.' 'Not so good, son, couldn't get off . . . then woke up again.' And best of all, considering the central heating pounds until our whole abode thumps and wheezes like a punctured drum, 'Did you hear that noise?'

That noise is always the boiler and at this time of year the heating is never off. Like some polar province, this house has seasons of its own. Winter here, if one were to measure it by the heating, is about 360 days long. It is an irony, hopefully not lost on future generations, that climate change was caused in part by people trying to keep their house's temperature the same.

Ecology apart, I have sympathy for the boiler as it struggles to do as it is asked. It is a domestic unit doing industrial labour, and it sounds like it. I find fellow feeling as it clanks towards its doom in service of other declining systems. The plumbing here is so old that the pipes are subject to 'kettling', a persistent thump and clang which is particularly pronounced in the vicinity of the boiler. Happily, my room is right next to it.

Every couple of years men are invited to the house to solve the problem and, after charging several hundred pounds, explain there is nothing much that they can do. Sleeping in my room then is like trying catch a nap in a goblin mine, find forty winks on the footplate of the Flying Scotsman or curling up in hell's belfry for a snooze.

So, yes, I will have heard 'that noise' and every other, and could map out each snore and toilet visit besides, since I too have been awake most of the night. Our sleepless situation will then resolve itself as the day unfolds into a patchwork of equally competitive and furiously defended napping.

When it does, occasionally, fall quiet at night, silence brings another issue. I have been woken so often now by the cries or operatic bronchial improvisations of one or both my parents that, like a new mother, I have evolved a hypersensitive reaction to the slightest noise. When things are tough here I'm not sure one ever properly sleeps at all. Lest this cultivate undue sympathy I should confess that being woken up by – and actually responding to – sounds of apparent distress, are two different things entirely.

You can play 'Are they coughing or dying?' all night long if you can live with the guilt, and apparently I can. Sometimes when I hear them call my name my first reaction is to wish it all away. Then I respond.

'What's an algorithm?' asks Mum this morning, shaking the newspaper with the vigilant air that signals the intrusion of a new phrase.

'It's like a machine that guesses what you want.'

'Can we get one?'

*

I make Dad his breakfast more out of expediency than necessity; he moves so slowly it is painful to watch him do this stuff alone. Not as painful as it is for him. His greatest ailments are unseen: COPD, diabetes, extensive arthritis, assorted rheumatic disorders, prostate cancer and ongoing complications from what we know now were a series of heart attacks that called me home nine months ago.

Since then he has made remarkable progress, not least by staying alive. After a few abortive bedside goodbyes and more than a month in hospital he carefully cast aside a pessimistic prognosis and a walking frame, embraced the complexities of catheterization and now enjoys, if that's the word, a tremendous quantity of drugs and a small measure of independence.

That measure is everything. Though living at home, he is a kind of Frankenpensioner, animated and sustained by outside forces, an array of tech, pharma and family that keep this being, so much of the previous century, participant in the present day. In recent years this declared functionality has been enabled only by his annexing of my mother as a kind of vassal state. He depends on her. My return and then her illness have slid the baton to me. My being here keeps them here and certain conversations at arm's length. If my fortunes were to change, they might be out of luck and perhaps the house. There seems no risk of that right now, but whatever it is we have here, it can't last. For the moment their mortality and my mental health appear to have eloped together. Nothing makes sense but we press on.

*

It's good that Dad's not in hospital but we still go there a lot, and parts of it come out to us. District nurses, practice nurses and even actual doctors. I have been medicalized by proximity over the last nine months. The processes and their prose are as infectious as any condition. I now speak catheter and kidney function. I am fluent in phlegm and several subdialects of drizzling shit. If you wanted to organize a heist at the local hospital I am that character in the movie who could lead you through it in darkness and, if need be, pretend to be a doctor.

Movies are a thing for me and Dad. He wanted to be an actor once and before the heyday of commercial aviation his ships carried some of the greats to and from America. I became aware early on that actors and writers were to be revered. Although if they were poor tippers or ill-mannered then this was never forgotten. We used to go the pictures together. And yet part of cinema's almost undue influence over me might have been that I grew up watching many films alone, here in the room where he now does the same. Meanwhile I think in movies, retreat into movies and even worked on some. My clearest moment of filial pride was when I called Dad to tell him I had met Clint Eastwood, only for thirty seconds, admittedly, but as those famous eyes narrowed on me my first thought was of the Old Man.

That was years ago, back in the mere matinee of old age. Here in the late show I help Dad sit down and get our breakfast on. I make Mum a cup of tea while he spoons up the blueberries and low-cholesterol yoghurt which are supposed to offset a lifetime of rationing, red meat and libation.

'I'm going to need more tissues,' he tells me.

'What are you planning?' I ask him, not really wanting an answer.

'We're running out.'

I check by his chair in the living room. There is indeed an empty box, but it is balanced on five full boxes so he can reach it without stretching.

'You don't need more tissues, you need a higher side table,' I suggest.

'No, no, no!'

He shakes his head and scowls as though his life depends on this insane arrangement, which for all I know, it does.

*

I go upstairs to Mum, pausing briefly to do a pull-up on the parallel banisters installed by the council's occupational therapy squad months ago.

I think about getting fit, but I am as delusional in that regard as I was when I raced up and down this staircase as a child.

Mum's room is much as it ever was. Neat, bookish and

warm. As is she. I used to think she looked like the Queen on pound notes. Now they're long gone but she and the Queen remain. The curtains are closed and her eyes barely open when I come in. I have no memories of Mum being ill like this. She snapped her ankle some years back, has bones brittle as breadsticks and suffered a mini-stroke but appeared spiritually undiminished by such setbacks. She seems to me a natural old person, taking even the hardest changes in her uneven, shrinking stride. Until now. No doubt I have tinted vision in this regard. She can complain with the best of them, though not to me so much. She and my sister have a singularly dysfunctional discourse in that respect. I get the complaints about the complaining; somehow this all works out.

At least, for me. My sister was the first to leave the nest and our hometown and the first to come back. She has spent the thirty years since then living down the road from our parents. Few big city lights for her. Instead a drip feed of them ageing, not getting along, getting along, helping, and needing help. She has worked the battlements here for decades, raised children and weathered her own divorce. A former primary school teacher, she has a kind of feral foresight for disaster, as though the whole world was a loose infant running into the road. She is a seasoned, if shell-shocked, soldier. I have deeper reserves, maybe, for this stage of our ride, having done largely as I pleased wherever I liked for the last three decades, even if I am surprised by how unhappy this left me.

Our brother is a more mercurial figure with a remarkable flair for raising havoc and money. Cars that cost more than houses driven into trees. That kind of thing. He is thus a worry in his own right but also tremendously effective, at large in the world and not yet reclaimed by the places that made us.

Meantime Mum has a way with words and an abstract and perceptive humour that can, on rare but memorable occasions, verge on cruelty. Seldom are her subjects in earshot or someone she knows. For anyone in the papers or on television it is open season. The appearance of Angelina Jolie, for instance, will raise a Pavlovian cry of –

'Don't adopt any more children!'

If on screen this will be accompanied by the standard –

'Ugh!!'

– applied to anyone deemed to have lurched up uninvited from the depths of her disdain. In that respect, her foes are legion. Amiable regional weatherman –

'Not him!'

Men with precise hair –

'Pretty boy!' And so on.

Once we knew each other's saints and sinners. Lately her metrics are beyond me. The last time we disliked the same thing in equal measure might have been Ace of Base's 1992 single 'All That She Wants'. Me on grounds of taste, her on the notion of wilful single parenthood espoused in the lyrics.

Now her vivacity and disdain have been consumed by shingles. The condition has condensed into a few red welts on her right arm, but the pain and anxiety that emanate from it are beyond all proportion to these outer signs. Hard to behold, though she does her best to mask it. She can't bring herself to read, which, for a book-a-week-and-two-newspapers-a-day person, is really saying something, even if she herself is largely silenced.

This contrast to her general wellness makes it more troubling, in part because it finds us both unprepared. She doesn't even want her tea today, which is most irregular. Dad, meanwhile, is simply surprised to have lived this long. It was never his intention. He was, I think, determined to smoke, drink and sit his way into an early grave, only to discover his body had other plans.

Our father's pessimistic slogans, 'I won't make old bones' (which he was still saying in his early eighties) and, 'You won't have to worry about me much longer,' echo like the broken campaign promises of some now entrenched regime. Harrowing as it can be when he takes a turn for the worse, it's expected. We know the terrain. Mum's pain is less familiar, and so plays harder on my mind.

Meals and Wheels

Having made it from the kitchen to the lounge unaided this morning, Dad is growing in confidence. It's been six weeks since he was last in hospital with pneumonia. Not content with reaching his armchair, he now feels like leaving the house. Driving, no less. Out for lunch, into the country. This should be cause for celebration. It's been weeks since we went anywhere.

I check the diary, just in case something is happening today. This small but vital volume which sits upon the breakfast bar is our family's holy book. Each year the numbers and addresses of those deemed important or simply still alive are hand-copied from one volume to the next. My parents were born in Lancashire but met in the mid Atlantic, working in the purser's office of an ocean liner. Perhaps these diaries offer some aspect of book-keeping labour that they can still take pride in. Beloved the system may be, functional it is not.

The pain and stiffness in Dad's hands has reduced his penmanship. A note from him looks like a confession wrought by torture. Mum's more measured hand has taken a baroque twist in later life that makes it harder than it ever was to understand. My own handwriting is awful, a fusion of impatience and broken bones. Sometimes we leave notes for one another, signs of life more than anything anyone can understand. We don't make sense, we make do.

While I scour the schedule, Dad has one of his outbreaks of practical morbidity.

'You know where everything is?' he asks.

This means the list of who to call and what to do when he passes. I have known this for so long now that I do tend to forget it. The clues are scattered: lists of hymns here, accountants' numbers there. Whatever happens and whenever it does, the diaries will be key, the Rosetta Stone of the whole household, and the book of the dead.

'Yes. I know what to do if you die,' I answer as I close the diary. 'Are you . . . definitely OK to drive?'

He doesn't answer, but he is now sporting his driving cap which means we will soon be under way, safely or not.

'Go,' says Mum. Glad to be alone, perhaps. A visit from the cleaner means she won't be, entirely, but I nevertheless glance up at her window as we leave.

Catching his breath in whatever is left of his lungs, Dad swings the motor around. I think again about learning to drive; I've been meaning to do it for thirty years. I had been meaning to do a lot of things. Pushing fifty and moving back in with my parents wasn't among them.

*

On the road, Dad is transformed. I'm happy to see him doing something well and enjoying it. It can take him breathless minutes just to open a letter. As we leave town I alternate between memories of childhood drives and the realization that, if he were to fall ill at the wheel, I might have to drag him free of the pedals and snatch the keys. This much I have deduced from movies.

In the event of an actual vehicular emergency I am like someone who has learnt English just from listening to the radio suddenly having to play competitive Scrabble: fucked.

Dad parks directly outside the front door of the pub. His disabled badge allows him to do this, and despite any number of available disabled spaces nearby, this is now what he does wherever he goes. The blue badge bandit: he's here, he's hungry and he's blocking your door.

The owner seats us by a roaring fire. Dad is pleased. His instinct for a warm place has become almost feline and since midsummer my parents have never quite been warm enough. This would probably still be the case if they moved to a smaller, more modern house at the heart of the sun.

He devours a plate of scallops, tells me he doesn't feel so good, then, as if struck by a bullet, he collapses.

I grab him in a way that feels therapeutic but more closely resembles a full nelson. I am oddly calm, or at least calmer than one might expect when imagining these types of situations. Also I've been 'here' before in recent years: small-hours emergency calls, sudden collapses, and a thousand times in my mind. A kind of well-drilled pessimism kicks in. I wouldn't call it courage. It feels more robotic, tense but almost numb somehow, while still another part of me enjoys the drama. After months of things feeling much the same, at least this is different. I signal to the owner to call an ambulance, ignore the stares of our fellow diners and ask plaintively in the Old Man's ear if he's all right, if he can hear me. Nothing.

I consider that if he has snuffed it, then this is not a bad way to go. Scallops, driving, pubs and fire. For what had threatened to be a long and perhaps undignified decline to have halted abruptly is no tragedy.

A paramedic arrives and we place my father across three chairs, like an extra in a stage illusion in which the seats will be removed and leave him suspended. Instead, an earthlier miracle: with his feet higher than his heart, Dad revives.

'Old people by the fire,' says the paramedic. 'Blood pressure plummets, they faint.'

Dad pukes so loudly the whole restaurant comes to a standstill.

'Not uncommon,' assures the paramedic.

'What shall I do with your lunch?' asks the pub landlord.

'I'll eat mine,' I tell him. Death is inevitable, yet it remains a sin to waste food.

The paramedic asks how we'll be getting home.

'I guess he shouldn't be driving?' I answer, through a mouthful of skate.

The paramedic shakes his head. Cab, then. Cabs from now on, maybe. If we ever go out again.

In the taxi I hold the orange plastic cracker box the landlord had given us for Dad to throw up into under his chin as he lolls beside me on the back seat. I'm not sure we've ever been in the back of a car together before. Ambulances, sure, but this is new for us. Perhaps we are bonding but I'm not sure how. We are both glad he hasn't had to go to hospital, albeit I suspect for different reasons.

He simply hates it. And as with most hates, what lies beneath is fear. For a man who spent his life travelling he is obsessed with being at home and dying there. Like some suburban pharaoh he has filled the place with souvenirs and prepared his burial chamber. Me, I know how long admissions take and don't have anything to read. I just don't want the rigmarole.

Besides, the pub is so far from the house that he would have ended up in an unfamiliar hospital. Longer journeys, fewer visits, all of that. And he has not been home long since his last hospitalization. So I hold my arm around him like a drunken friend, feeling nothing but curiosity at how little I do feel. What I thought was life has gone up in smoke like the fire in the pub. Including, it seems, my ability to be surprised. Are we callous or just protecting ourselves? What is a callous anyway, but a thing grown over a wound?

The cab driver is kind. They tend to be. He helps me get him inside. Dad is struggling to say something so I say it for him.

'Tip him?'

He nods. The Old Man is a big fan of the pay-off. I know it well. Money being what you can give if you can't be around. I pass the driver a fiver. Dad sinks into his chair and closes his eyes. Safely back in the pyramid, Pharaoh sleeps but makes no sound.

*

Mum takes the news of Dad's collapse calmly. There have been other 'turns', as she calls them, or 'vacant episodes', as they are known in the trade. It is a measure of human adaptability how quickly these things: attacks, collapses, ambulances and so on, become no big deal. Mum greets paramedics as calmly as she does the postman. We are getting better at this. Or perhaps today we are each too busy with our own pain. Either way, feeding time beckons.

In her illness Mum has come to like the things I used to as a kid. A mug of tomato soup. If she is feeling brave, a fish finger.

'I had forgotten about those!' she says when I suggest them.

I hadn't. Never stopped eating them. I was nutritionally immature long before it was fashionable.

If I told her comfort food was mainstream cuisine now I'm not sure she'd believe me. I like cooking it for her, though. It's fair trade. I have no idea what I am doing with my life except this. There is no bigger picture. Life is simply whatever goes down, I tell myself. Feeding the person who fed you when you were ill feels like a blessing. So far at least.

'What's this!?' Mum wants to know, holding something, on a downstairs mission.

It's a halogen light bulb, I explain.

'I almost put it in my mouth and ate it.'

Why?

'It was on the kitchen table.'

When so much of our world is vagary and mistakes, we are fortunate to have some good we can do. Still, I can't conceive of what this would be like if you disliked your parents or the reverse were true, or mutual. Or they didn't recognize you any more. Never mind the light bulbs.

Even our household's mild baggage is enough to bear. I make Mum soup, check Dad is still sleeping (he is, the plastic box for vomit empty and discarded by his side) and cook myself some pasta like the adult I pretend to be.

Tonight things are uncommonly quiet. Despite what you

might imagine, in the twilight years hush is hard to come by if anyone's awake. Our once demure and deferential household has been remixed by old age into a free-fire zone of profanity, fluids, flatulence and incredibly loud TV.

For years the most you would have heard here was a yawn. Now everything spoken is yelled. In the last nine months I've witnessed symphonies of farts that have lasted longer than many of our conversations, and simple conversations conducted at operatic volume, then repeated until there can be no doubt that yes it is Monday, or Tuesday, that yes Mum has her hearing aids in, or whatever else has been misheard or mis-said.

'Your parents fight,' one of the neighbours said to me, sadly, back in the summer.

No, I explained, that's just them talking. Or maybe just one of them on the phone.

The centre of this sonic confusion is the kitchen. Nutrition, medication, laundry – it all happens here. Adjoining it is a small bathroom, which adds to the fun. Although separated by double doors, my father is insistent on leaving these open (driven, according to my sister, by a fear of dying on the toilet like Elvis). This means that, to all intents and purposes, and certainly in terms of sound, the toilet is in the kitchen, too.

I have a lot of time for that small downstairs bathroom. As a teenager, it was there that I first confronted my reflection having lost my virginity. And it was there, not long afterwards, that I watched the nascent stubble on my face appear to ripple as I struggled with my first hit of LSD.

The tiny mirror that bore witness to these adolescent mile-stones is also a favourite of my father's. He likes to take it with him when he goes to hospital, so he can inspect the latest indignities that time has inflicted on his scalp and face.

'Why does he need it?' Mum will hiss on finding it gone again. I have tried giving him a different mirror, but he pines for the original.

The mirror business, like so many other seemingly innocuous things that, in a younger household, might submit to logic, will run and run. I have found it useful, when considering if and how to intervene in the everyday contretemps that permeate my parents' sixty-year marriage, to remember that one day, soon, there will be nothing to argue about and no one to argue with.

Meanwhile, the downstairs bathroom throws back vengeful echoes of my youthful escapades. On a good day, this means nothing more than Dad paying one of his catheter-emptying visits every hour or so. On less fortunate occasions, incontinence strikes and the scenes then are somewhere on the margins of agriculture, protest and performance art.

It is a very small space in which to operate, particularly when one must work around the victim of the latest indignity. Over time we have discovered that best practice is for the sufferer to remain where they are until the first stages of clean-up are done. When I snap on another pair of nitrile gloves (and if there is a single invention that makes all these things bearable, it is a box of nitrile gloves), I reflect that there is something to be said for a family that has entered a post-embarrassment culture. From divorce and depression to the details of digestion, all our intimacies are open now. In the room of furtive reflections, we finally have nothing to hide.

Sleeper Cell

3 November 2017

Things are back to what passes for normal; Dad moves slowly and Mum less.

'Do you want a scrambled egg?' I call up to her.

'I'm not in the bathroom!' she replies. Hearing aids evidently out of play this morning.

The car is recovered via a complex manoeuvre involving my brother and his brother-in-law, John, who is also a good friend of mine. By mid afternoon it is safely back in the garage, perhaps forever. Back in the house everyone is asleep again.

Sleep was always treasured here. When Dad came back from the ships I would be instructed to play quietly or elsewhere until he had got himself back on GMT. Much like now, the curtains would be drawn in the daytime, summer suns thwarted by orange drapes, giving the place a yellowish, digestive glow.

Years later, whenever I came home I would walk into the lounge and almost any discussion of the journey or the recent past would be met with –

'Why don't you go and have a lie-down?'

A suggestion to which I was and remain highly receptive.

Even now when there aren't things to do they are always urging me to sleep, like some hangover from infancy. This is how we roll as a family. With our eyes closed. It could all be much worse. I mean no slur on our conscious experiences here, but I have some great memories of when no one was awake.

'Did it matter?' Dad asked me once, years ago, about his not being around, working abroad. 'Did I do the right thing?'

I never knew any different and said so. It didn't bother me then. But then I wasn't divorced or getting old. Now my own emotional limitations and inclinations have wrought such trouble that I am not so sure. I don't feel ready to be certain, either. Some unfinished business simmers inside me and always did, perhaps. Life is different in the rear-view than through the windscreen. For now, it seems safer to lie down than to ask questions. Objects in the mirror may be closer than they appear.

Sleep, then, is our squad goal. When my parents are unconscious I get a clear sense of relief, of a job well done. When we sleep, no one is hungry, hot, cold, uncomfortable, confused or annoyed. 'Nature's soft nurse,' as Shakespeare called it, is kinder than I could ever be, yet we have become reliant on doctors for our supply.

I forget when I realized my dad had a repeat prescription for powerful tranquillizers. It feels like fifteen years or so, back in the benign lowlands of his early seventies – turf I no longer consider to be old age.

I was emerging then, belatedly, from an indulgent narcotic phase which had lasted since my late teens. I would frequently purloin his pills in subtle quantities to 'take the edge off' this or that. Sometimes this or that was everything. I have been described convivially and diagnosed officially as depressed, but sadness often seemed to me to be a reasoned response to an unreasonable condition: being alive. Not always, though. 'What do YOU have to be upset about?' I would ask myself, if someone else wasn't already asking. Now at least my moods have material grounds. Despite largely cleaning up from prescribed and recreational drugs, I still deploy bits of my father's cache at the end of whatever I deem to be a difficult day. And I will take the sandman over my solicitor or further self-reflection any time.

At least, I imagine the quantities of pills purloined are subtle. For all I know this might be another of our silent bonds. Perhaps he knows but says nothing. In a way I hope so. I can go without, but the Old Man goes into an anticipatory tailspin (like most of us, he is more panicked by the foreseen than the experienced) whenever supplies are low.

I say this, but I am in fact the same. I don't take them every night and when I do I deal in fragments, but at the idea of having none to hand, I break into a sweat. Between the heating and the heartaches and the desire to hear nothing at all, I am increasingly reliant on them. My own doctor gave me some that are absolutely stupefying, which I don't relish or risk any more.

The economy of bedtime has been complicated by Mum's arrival on the sickness scene. Undone by her illness, she neither sleeps well nor devours the days as she once did. Proud of nearing her tenth decade on nothing more than a daily aspirin, the moment she asked for some of 'Dad's tablets' was doubly significant since it betrayed a depth to her discomfort she might not otherwise express. Soon there are so many drugs changing hands here it is like an ancient, all-white version of *The Wire*.

Dad is more than happy to include her in the hustle. Me, less so, since I have a deeper fear about us running out than I can afford to admit to. Also, these twilight lives are in the balance. A pill here or there can make all the difference. If I confess what's afoot to one doctor, will they undo the tacit overprescribing of the other and bring the whole house of narco-cards down? Besides, for now, it works.

At night I break Dad's pills, keep half and hand a piece to Mum along with a lecture about addiction. I had a dealer myself once who did the same thing. Dad seems keen to induct her into his pharma-army. He, I think, ran short of strategies to soothe her long ago. Pills, though, pills he can do. He even comes into her room to drop them off. Since my sister got married and surrendered her bedroom to Mum our parents have slept staunchly apart. In the forty-odd years since, I have barely seen him in there.

'Careful, now,' I say as I lay out the tablets.

She doesn't answer but her look, I think, says, 'Please don't tell me what to do when I have so little distance left to run.'

When the principals are safely horizontal I repair to my lair and watch *Narcos*. I can relate to Pablo Escobar right now. Although I note that, despite murdering hundreds, he never ran drugs to his own mother. I make a mental note to pitch a series set on our landing to Netflix, turn out the lights and take my taste of oblivion.

5 November 2017

A quick phone call, late morning. I hear Dad stumble through condolences and realize what this is. I sit with my sorrow then go to his side. Bill, another one of their friends, has died. Not unexpected, but still. Theirs is a dwindling band. They are now the last surviving couple they know. A peculiar kind of victory. Sometimes I can imagine how they feel, but this, the death of almost every friend, I cannot fathom. Dad is not one for signifying emotion. I have only once seen him cry and that was partly down to me and I am in no hurry to see it again. I say –

'I'll go upstairs and tell her.'

Mum is in bed, neither awake nor asleep exactly. I share what's happened. She tells me stories about their friend. I have heard them all before but lie down beside her as she recalls his eating habits.

'He was very precise. You should have seen him take a fish off the bone, it could take forever. Slim, but he could put some food away . . . very good company, even when he went blind.'

I have my own memories of him. His family were our neighbours before we moved here. Early childhood. Their youngest son my first real friend. Bill was a good photographer. He took a black-and-white picture of me that I still have. It must be about 1975 and I am laughing. Consumed by it. I look as happy as a kid can be.

Now I seem sadder than my folks. They are steeped in all this. Seasoned, practically professionals of passing. So many people they know have died now that it happens less these days. The Omaha Beach years have been and gone. Only stragglers survive. I go to my room and cry. About what, I don't even know. The queue of sorrows seems unending.

Silence at Court

If sleep is treasured here, quiet is the next best currency. Having already hit the silence jackpot via deafness, Mum is less concerned, whereas my father craves to conduct his restless house to stillness like some miser of sound.

'I can hear the television!' he yells down from his bedroom, when I am trying to watch it after hours.

This is odd, since when he has it on you could hear it from any nearby town. I know better than to fight things here with logic, though. Hush here is not just capital, but also the final goal. I long for my own place, somewhere I can throw my own silence around.

When happy or reflective and not watching some deafening film, Dad will stare out of the window or close his eyes and say simply –

'So quiet.'

He grew up in an industrial town and the ships he worked on were ever-droning things. That he has made it to a suburban cul-de-sac defended from others by distance and dense foliage is, more than I can grasp, perhaps, the realization of some deep dream. But quiet here, like cleanliness, can never last.

Beside the boiler, chief disruptor of our idyll is the front door. Its heavy knocker might be better suited to a larger property, a castle or a missile silo. Certainly the effect upon the front room when its denizens are not expecting it, or asleep, is like cannon fire. In so far as their frames allow, both my parents will respond to the door like resting firemen, rousing to an unknown crisis.

Depending on where I am hiding at the time, I yell that I will get it. But by then an argument will have started between them, although these things are less arguments now than call-and-response mantras: 'Who is it?' 'I don't know.' 'What is it?' 'THE DOOR!' A duet between two climbers ascending into fog. If I don't act fast, or just can't be bothered, one of them will lurch unsteadily toward the portal. Each knock a potential heart attack, each trip a possible fall.

Prime Numbers

7 November 2017

I am quietly navigating the downstairs of the house since *a)* silence is the goal, and *b)* if they can't hear you they tend not to ask for anything. Despite having trained intensively to get about the house unnoticed as a child, I do occasionally breathe or rustle. Having zeroed in on my existence, Dad calls me into his domain, the front room – as hot as Saudi Arabia but with stricter rules about what's on television.

I enter braced for instructions. Coming in here is like Bond being summoned by M. You leave with a mission.

'Jeff Bezos,' announces Dad admiringly, 'richest man in the world!'

He leans forward from the chair in which he will spend the rest of the day and perhaps his life and offers me the paper. I refuse it, saying, 'I know,' and immediately dislike myself for doing so.

Dad seems hurt that I don't want to read about Bezos and his money, but it's because I am beginning to get a sense of just how much of Bezos's money was once my father's.

Though he loves an entrepreneur, my father hails from a

vanished land of unionized labour and pensions. The same pension that keeps the house at the approximate temperature of the palm house at Kew all year round ensures a steady stream of Bezos's foot soldiers to our door. I say door, but the daily, sometimes hourly Amazon deliveries can materialize anywhere within a 20-metre radius of the house, depending on the duress and the demeanour of the courier.

From the absurd: a single bottle of lemonade (Me: 'I go to the shops!' Him: 'I was thirsty'); to the absurdly wrapped: a walking stick packaged like a running machine; to the poignant succession of balms, salves and medical ephemera, the deliveries form a steady cardboard tide.

The council have cut the recycling collection back to once a fortnight and there is more here than any mortal wheelie bin can cope with. Indoors, where my father pounds a rubberized wand into his Samsung tablet ordering yet more of Jeff's treasure, it is 2017. At the side of the house the bins are overflowing and it's like the strikes of 1979. I take a Stanley knife to another piece of cardboard, stuff it into the recycling and curse the innovations in healthcare and home delivery that have come to shape my days.

I used to play tennis up against this wall. Now I work out latent violence with a blade. I carve up another cardboard rival and hope the neighbours cannot see.

Despite a flurry of Amazon-related gags – 'All this comes from South America?' – Mum has relapsed into mostly quiet annoyance as my father stirs the world to pointless action from his chair. A certain dark humour is essential for our survival, but one must deploy it carefully. As death is proximal – their friends die, hospital doctors take me to one side each time they let him go – we must make light of it, but also recognize that to do so is to run on heavy fuel. What makes for catharsis one day can crush you the next. I bite my lip and mutter. I think we all do.

Having shopped for us all, and then just them till she was no longer able, Mum's awareness of the cause-and-effect chain behind bringing something to the table is keener than Dad's will ever be. That he has in his dotage secured a mastery of technology that effectively cuts her out of the loop forms but another strand in the bonds and resentments that sustain them.

When he hovers over his next purchase with his special screen-stabbing stick, I sense that down the thread of history our common ancestor took similar aim against a mammoth. Every pointless purchase is primal in its way. When he is gone, if there is still money, perhaps I will journey to the actual Amazon and throw the special stick into the river in case Jeff Bezos's hand should rise from the waters to reclaim it.

With Mum upstairs, if I'm not in, Dad must attend to Jeff's legions. This is entirely fair enough since what arrives are mostly things he has summoned, and which will benefit him alone. Assuming, of course, that he has ordered what he thinks he has.

Sometimes what turns up is quite unfathomable and he will deny having bought it. It could be that his memory is worsening, or the more amenable if mischievous interpretation, that he is simply trolling us all.

Spontaneous action is not my father's thing, so I am surprised to come back from the shops and find he has taped a square of the (abundant) cardboard to the striker where the knocker meets the front door. Like an assassin silencing his weapon. But to what end?

My sister reaches instinctively for the most Machiavellian interpretation.

'It's so he doesn't have to get up and answer it!'

I counter that he has that option anyway, and that if we must apportion blame for this amendment, it is that it will have been made in service of the household's sacred and related goals: sleep and silence. We settle on some combination of both. Dad flanks our cynicism with an assertion of selflessness.

'It's so your mother isn't disturbed.'

The truth lies somewhere in the middle of all these motives, I suspect. If Dad imagines something vital has arrived, drugs perhaps, or a DVD of a movie he already has a DVD of and which is freely available online, then he will do some Lazarus/ Lourdes manoeuvre, rise from his chair and do his stooped best to make it to the door on time. This, then, is how I have come to square this daily madness in my soul: Jeff Bezos is Dad's physio. At least until the real one calls.

Lounge Lizards

8 November 2017

The telephone is a kind of door in miniature in so far as it can shatter the sacred semi-silence, but also deliver the high bounty of decrepitude the Old Man craves. Doctors, children, chemists, restaurants (when sufficiently mobile), we all respond to him this way.

Unlike the door which thumps like ordnance, the phone rings at a pitch which can elude Mum completely. Dad then is the default receptionist at this office of dysfunction and so if I am out or otherwise engaged it falls to him to keep the rogues at bay.

The volume of hoax calls, telemarketing, and pernicious aural spam directed at an elderly household is phenomenal. I have worked in frantic offices where things were quieter. It matters not which directories you exit or what preferences you set, somewhere in the world in some extrajudicial circle of hell, there are rooms full of underpaid young people calling the houses of older people in a bid to redistribute whatever wealth is perceived to be there.

Conversely, the nuisance calls can generate some laughs and

even fellow feeling. It is merciful that my parents have their wits about them to the point where they can mostly tell the wheat from the chaff with this stuff. Nothing major has been bought, surrendered or remortgaged. Yet.

When Mum does answer the phone my sympathies are largely with the caller. She has all the time in the world for you to fruitlessly explain yourself to her. You presumably have targets, dreams and plans of your own. There can only be one winner here. And she can't even hear you.

Likewise the perished possibilities of my own life mean I can stay on the phone as long as you like. I have elevated some of these conversations to the level of hostage negotiation. Some callers are so persistent that, as with resourceful junkies, you cannot but feel heartache as to what all that potential might have been.

'You should hang up or this will never end,' is a phrase that gets results, I find.

*

Dad answers a call. I can hear him in the bathroom (a scato-logical radar station on a par with its downstairs cousin) as he improvises a series of wild, brusque excuses: 'No . . . I can't, not today . . . not up to it . . . no,' over the phone. This continues in what I think of, perhaps cruelly, as his special 'weak old man' tone, before he hangs up, rudely. I know there is only one person this can be. I close in on the Old Man and make like I don't know what is happening. I have seen enough cop shows to know the key to a successful case is to have your felon self-incriminate. I open with a benign –

'Who was that, then?'

But before Dad can answer I am reminded of why I wouldn't have made a good policeman. The instance between the appearance of my good cop and my bad cop is too slender for anyone's good. I would be surprised if my dad didn't know this since he is – *drum roll* – exactly the same.

'That was the physio, wasn't it? He wants to come and help us, but you told him to go away.'

'I don't feel well.'

Fair enough, given his recent struggle, but the physio has been on my father's trail for months and regardless of his actual health my father still eludes him. 'He doesn't want to get better,' my sister will say, and when this seems true to me as well there is a sudden shift inside. I find I am equipped with an anger so complete that it must have been assembled long ago.

'Bullshit,' I say, as he absconds slowly across the landing. 'You can barely move because you don't try to move, and when someone wants to help you move you turn away.'

He makes a noise like a cornered animal. A small one at that. So I was right.

That I have extracted a silence from which guilt can be inferred from an eighty-seven-year-old man in a towel takes some of the shine off things. I release him into the community (his bedroom) and call the physio back.

'Hello again,' he says.

He knows the number and my voice. I have promised him progress before, but recalcitrant elderly folk are nothing new to him. This being the NHS, he exudes a fatalistic calm.

I admire him for even picking up the phone.

I apologize for my father: 'He's not himself,' although in truth swerving physical activity is quintessentially him.

Even so, to waste a man's time, to add to our burden through his own immobility, these are not his intentions even if they are the outcomes.

'Call back with some dates. I'll try again,' says the physio. The question is, will Dad?

My sister's approach, which is more of an ambush or air strike, is more consistently confrontational. She is a Pilates instructor with many elderly clients. Old people sitting still is anathema to her. Add untold Freudian baggage into this and her versus my dad in the lounge becomes the kind of contest Don King would promote. The Brawl in the Shawl. The Melee by the Tellee.

This manifests chiefly through her loud repetition of emotive phrases and bleak mottoes uttered at speed, in the manner of an American agricultural auctioneer or a Dancehall MC. 'Use it or lose it!' 'Atrophy!' 'Hip!' 'Incontinence!' 'Bedridden!' 'Death!' Plenty of shock, not much awe. You just tap out or flee (though Dad has neither option). Which is a shame since she is, underneath all that reflex and technique, usually right.

The Old Man just sits there and says absolutely nothing. He will dependably take things up a notch by closing his eyes and turning his head away. As though the end itself were preferable to your presence. The result is a spiritual filleting of the assailant. You wilt inside.

If I told her about the physio business she would be outraged. So I must pep talk the Old Man about his mobility.

When the urge to punish him has subsided I close in. He's perched on his bed and closes his eyes, as per, perhaps imagining that the temperature of the room will prevent me from loitering. But I am not to be dissuaded. Even if I have to come back in a thong.

'Think about how good it is not being in hospital, and how many times they've helped you out of there.'

He nods. We both know we've been unreasonable. Still I continue –

'We can't do everything for you here, and they're sending a man to the house who will show you how to use your limbs again . . .'

'I know, I know . . .'

When we have navigated one another's defences what follows is amazing, though often at risk of being overwhelmed by my regret that we can't do this more often. When he accepts a lecture I want to weep for all we *could* be saying. He is embarrassed by his behaviour, means no harm. Me neither.

Though he looks every one of his years I just don't see him as 'old', somehow. He is just and always my father. It is an image that can obscure the simple realities. But then I knew the image of him over and above the individual in some ways. He would send postcards from wherever he was working. I still feel closer to words than to people at times. But we are close now. I breathe in his room, the magic, myriad odour of ownership we all somehow create. I used to come in here and sense him when he was away. One of the embedded ironies of caring is that emotional proximity to others can also make us less sensitive to their pain. Sometimes we are too close to be of comfort. I notice the radiator in his room is leaking water onto the carpet. I go to turn the valve.

'Don't touch that!' says Dad. 'It's exactly right.'

Dad coughs as he looks out of the window. COPD leaves him breathless from what should be effortless, even at his age. Every mealtime is a mountain. Sometimes when he stands he feels dizzy enough to fall. Falling is the great fear, he knows what that means. The notion that someone might come and make you do exercises equates in this mindset with danger. That it might also be an opportunity is something of a hard sell. When I am tired I think, add another forty years to this, myself, how might that feel? And he has deeper sorrows than I could ever fathom.

My father was his mother's only child and she died before he ever knew her. More than his physical pain or maybe deeply rooted in it, this, I think, might be what governs him inside. With my own mother still vivid and beside me I fight not to judge him for what he has become to fill such absence in his life. He gave to me what he couldn't have himself. A mother, siblings, space and higher learning. I cannot stand here and inflict on him the privilege of my pride. Not that that stops me trying. I sit beside him. We sort of hug.

'Can I have a biscuit?' he asks, and our moment of empathy and timeless wisdom crumbles like a rusk.

His appalling diet is as sure a driver of his ill health as his progressive immobility. Admission of one tragic habit followed by reversion to another is classic Dad. We break like fighters from the clinch. We have acknowledged our frailties. We have tried. Despite residual inner battles I fetch this ailing diabetic another biscuit. You do what you can, and then give in. I have never had a dog or a baby but have noted that the lecture/ biscuit cycle appears to be much the same in those arenas. Nonetheless, I book a visit with the physio and eat a biscuit myself on the sly.

Who's the Daddy?

9 November 2017

You can't give the mobility lecture then sit still yourself, not that I am inclined to. The urge to just lie down and give up is offset by a drive to get out of this house if it's at all possible. When everyone seems OK, I tend to flee. Nowhere special, just not here.

Sometimes on foot, sometimes on an old pushbike I borrow from my sister which collapses like some clown's accessory with dependable regularity and dumps me to the ground. Sometimes I get the bus to town.

While the house I grew up in seems eerily the same, the city has devoured, rebuilt and reimagined itself to something almost unrecognizable. Bombed heavily and rebuilt hastily, it is an odd mixture of medieval remnants and fast-outmoded modern mistakes. The place is very much an old person, slapping on the warpaint to appear vital while the world's momentum moves away. It takes more than an Apple Store to fight this level of decay.

The key, of course, is people. I have memories to fill the gaps where the terrain has changed but I am blessed by how many allies I still have here. Without others to turn to all this, my life, might be a crushing errand. My friends are busy in the days, so I head to the library for a change of scene. I came here to write as a teenager with a head full of dreams. This wasn't one of them.

The city library doubles as a Citizens' Advice bureau. In addition to those who simply come here to keep warm this draws in a stream of people who have no idea what to do or who to turn to. Those in the throes of eviction, redundancy, deportation and the mentally ill. Quiet it isn't, but like hospital, it offers the gift of context. A couple of hours there and self-pity is gone.

I had not long ago applied and been turned down for a job as a librarian, which had annoyed me. But I see now there is a lot more to it than being well read. I take out my laptop and approach my inbox like an exploded bomb. No sign of work and plenty of divorce. The person who knew who he was or what he did seems like some long-lost friend. Someone sets off the fire alarm. I catch the bus home.

When I get in there are cries of confusion from the living room. The house is like an app; you can swipe left when you come through the front door, and get yourself together in the kitchen, or turn right and face the facts. I make a right . . .

What strikes me first is not so much that Mum is out of bed, but that Dad is at the far side of the lounge from where he sits. I'm not sure I've seen him down this end of the room since the late 1990s. What's also noticeable is that he is on his hands and knees, apparently bowing to the television. He repeats a phrase, faintly.

'I don't know . . . I don't know . . .'

One hears a lot about patriarchy these days, but I am mostly sweeping out the ashes of such.

For a moment I think maybe the oft-discussed and heavily guarded marbles of the old man's mind have finally departed. It is such an odd sight that I wonder also if he is somehow possessed, even if I don't, ordinarily, believe in such things. Most days it would take something supernatural just to get him out of his chair.

Mum looks despairing. And then she says in the special hiss she believes renders her inaudible to whoever she's discussing –

'He's on the phone to the TV people.'

Suddenly, everything is clear. He is bent double trying to fix the satellite receiver and has a phone to his ear.

I take the phone and help him up. The person on the line is trying to sell him an expanded TV package. I explain that he is no longer listening, that I am his son.

'Put Daddy back on the phone,' says the man in the call centre.

I freeze at this. My dad has never been known as 'Daddy', and we are not about to start now.

As I ferry him back to his seat, I figure out what has gone down, and it is in these kinds of mindless crises that I really come into my own. With mum's deafness it is essential that the TV has subtitles, or it must be at a volume that could destroy a passing bird.

As it is, it is often so loud they should be in high-vis jackets. Anyway, the subtitles went off and the Old Man has had to call the service provider to turn them back on. Somehow this has *a)* not been accomplished, and *b)* evolved into an attempt to make him pay even more for watching television.

I press the buttons that reinstate the subtitles. I have done this before; I will do it again. It's part of the elderly care territory. You become their short-term memory. A portable hard drive. Meanwhile:

'Where is Daddy?'

'Please don't say "Daddy",' I ask.

'Daddy wants the expanded package,' insists the call-centre caller.

'I'm an idiot,' says Dad, ruefully.

I promise him he's not. He seems unconvinced.

'Turn this up!' yells Mum, even though the subtitles are back on. It's an advert.

'Where is Daddy!?'

He's really going for it now, this desperate, distant salesman.

'Daddy doesn't want to talk to you any more,' I say.

And Daddy nods. I live in part for these small moments of consensus. As the television spells out dialogue that's already old, I hang up the phone.

After such interventions, embarrassment and futility can hang heavy in the elderly air. But we know well how to move on in this house. We get the kettle on.

*

Our tea ceremony is reassurance. Three mugs mean we are all surviving, have appetites and functioning fingers. Three mugs say all is well. The moment between the first rumble of the boiling water and the off-click of the kettle switch becomes a holy instant of dependable calm.

When I deliver the drinks I try and stay and share the moment rather than just running to another room, but this depends what's on TV. Sometimes the wall of warmth and sound is just too much and one must back away reluctantly, like a firefighter driven from a blaze. It was freezing in town so for now I enjoy the heat and settle down.

Their latest TV has devoured a corner of the room. When we moved in, forty-odd years ago, TV was something to be slightly ashamed of, at least in terms of my mother's aspirations. A device of mirth and music, but also moral turpitude and social doom. Ours had a wooden cabinet; you could draw a shutter around so you couldn't see the screen. It was still blatantly a television set, though, you wouldn't want to disguise that entirely, so much as signify you weren't in thrall to it. Not that there was that much on. My mother supervised the spread of tech into the household like a customs inspector, which was wise as my dad would otherwise buy almost anything invented. We were the last people I knew to have a video recorder but remain the only ones to have a trouser press.

Now all such constraints are gone, it's a free-for-all; they will take whatever they can get. From ionizers to light-switch timers, all aligned in full pagan subordination to the Panasonic monolith TV in the corner. Tech-henge. An upside to Dad not getting to the shops is that he might not be aware you can get an even bigger screen. As it is, it is hard enough to convince him not to buy a sound bar, given the existing wattage could make a dub reggae sound system seem undersized.

By fate and disposition this room is the Old Man's world. This is the last arena. Here, sitting down, is his final stand.

Who's the Daddy?

With his trusty, deaf sidekick they apply themselves to a world it must seem tough to understand. It is some road, from the late 1920s to this reality. It is never long before something comes on screen to blow their minds. Though seldom what you might expect.

Tonight's issue is an old one. They get the 'wrong' local news and weather. Some quirk of transmission or geography means that certain bulletins emanate from a town they do not recognize. The news anchor ('Who's *he*!?') sits by a photo of a bridge we have never crossed ('Where's *this*?'). It's as if they have been physically transported to some unwanted and reviled dimension. I have enough time on my hands to image-search it and confirm that, indeed, this is information leaking in from the next county. Indignant frowns on already wrinkled brows thicken and multiply.

The wrong news. Sure, we can do the cognitive dissonance on the national stuff and the refugees in the Mediterranean. As the world burns we know exactly when to sigh. But when it comes to people just up the motorway? Fuck them, their traffic, their sports achievements and June brides. Even the worst middle-distance tragedies yield only impatience.

'Gerroff,' they mutter at the screen together, as though TV were the music hall or some presumptuous lover.

All is forgiven with the onset of *Coronation Street*. It is one of their peculiar rituals that my dad will summon my mother, often as not 'pottering' elsewhere, as the show commences, bellowing her first name repeatedly and yelling '*Street!*' as though it were a dog or a kestrel, until she is safely back on the sofa. That he has at his disposal and understands the technology to pause the show or record it is not the point. This is ceremonial. Soldiers marching outside a palace where no power resides. In the end you become a tourist in your own life. Checking the familiar sights are there.

Another beloved and reliable recurrence is the show *Foyle's War*. Even the whispered dialogue of espionage belts out of the set like a speech from Nuremberg. I tend to leave them to it at this point. The programme appears to have been on daily for the last fifteen years. 'Longer than the real war', is one of our shared jokes about this. When we have a common aside we make the most of it. These things are code for love. And remembrance.

We Few

If November moved any slower you might think it was in reverse. Remembrance Sunday, however, is hard to miss, as this provides the cue for things to get loud. Before the guns fall silent Dad views the memorial services and any prior documentary footage at a volume and a level of reverence reserved for this alone.

I have turned the room next door— the 'dining room', where we hardly ever dined, into an office, where I hardly ever work. I arrange myself on the ornate but painful chairs and try to compose an email, but the vibrations from Whitehall and Flanders next door are making this impossible.

It behoves my generation to be happy that inconvenience constitutes the greater obstacle to our well-being than the muddy, martial deaths that faced those who came before us. I appreciate that I am already twice as old as someone who might have been writing home from the front lines of either of this country's defining conflicts, and that heavy metal and acid house have numbed my senses more than Howitzers and chlorine. But still . . .

The volume of the TV rattles through a silver tea caddy which contains a letter of thanks from troops billeted in my great-grandmother's house. The ghosts are as restless this morning as they are revered. I beat my own retreat and take the laptop to the bedroom.

Vietnam documentaries have replaced *Narcos* as my escapist weapon of choice. Both offer the spectacle of young men sent to their death for shitty reasons or none at all. It is an odd, perhaps quite male thing to fixate on conflicts you have played no part in and wonder what you might have done. Is Dad (just too young to serve in the Second World War) wondering if it might have been better to go out fighting, just as I am up here wondering if it might have been better to have fought at all?

The Analogue Alamo

Dad isn't about to drive anywhere so I head out for the newspaper. Going to buy it had become a daily battle for my parents, one of many apparently unnecessary errands that nevertheless kept them moving and sane.

The newsagent that delivered, which was also a post office, is long gone, replaced by a chain supermarket that offers none of the services beloved by the older generation. Posting, newsprint, letters. How many forgotten households use these to survive? It is another of later life's rebuttals when even the high street wants nothing to do with you. The neighbourhoods are changing and there are very few businesses that seem to want you alive. The message from the abandoned storefronts is: Go home. Give up. Live online or die.

Free from the analogue Alamo, I march up the hill. A good thing to do anyway. I breathe cold, fresh air and step carefully across the beds of moss that coat the shaded pavements all year long. Neither of my folks could make it up here now. In forty years I don't think I have even seen Dad try. He prefers to drive. The more Mum moved the less he walked anywhere.

She joined a local ramblers' group, he stayed inside. Now his legs have taken the hint. I pray to be different. Grateful as the gradient nags. Tendons tested. Burning thighs.

I head past houses my friends have long since left behind. Past dense green rhododendrons hiding yellow rental bikes, shipped from China, tossed away inside. The last petrol station before the motorway is the nearest place to buy a newspaper. I used to come up here as a kid and use the toilet, just for something different to do. They since got rid of the toilet. Much to my father's annoyance. Not that he comes out this way these days, but he judges the state of the world from such decisions. I believe he may be onto something.

On the forecourt, tanks are filled for longer journeys. I grab a paper from the stands and head inside, where the man behind the counter has a smile so vivid and reliable I have known it cut through blues I thought were some permanent aspect of my person. I am becoming dependent on these kinds of things. If he isn't here I feel compromised. Bereft. Am I coming for the paper at all?

*

Back home, my sister has been and dropped off another paper. This happens a lot. When Dad is in hospital I have known us as a group to have purchased five copies of the same title. We are keeping newsprint alive. Newspaper is only a part of the problem here. When the planet withers into flame or ice or famine, this house will have played its part with pride.

As a threat to the world's forests we must rank somewhere close to hardwoods, palm oil and strip mining. My parents' quest for paper in one form or another is unending. After hot air and warm water the things we consume the most of here are tissues and paper towels.

My father's hands have succumbed to some hybrid of gout and arthritis that no one can quite diagnose but which robs him of dexterity and yields constant pain. Mealtimes then are a carnival of mishaps. To limit the laundry outcomes and in a dignity-preserving manoeuvre which, like many such exercises, is far from dignified, my father fashions a patchwork breastplate made of several paper towels. These are tucked into his clothing or under his chin in a series of pre-flight checks that cannot be omitted before eating can begin.

What he does tend to omit if the paper towels are not laid out and ready as he sits, slowly and painfully, at the end of the table, are the rules of basic politeness or sentence construction. He calls out to remedy the situation –

'Towels!'

– as if he was helping someone give birth. Something I'm fairly sure he hasn't done since the moment of my conception.

This method of asking for things: noun, followed, possibly, by your name, is not conducive to a happy home. That someone whose well-being consumes so much of one's day chooses to communicate trivia in the manner of one managing a crisis rather than causing it, is something of a wind-up. It is ever the small things that break us. At these moments, which are often, I think of Chekhov's line about how any idiot can thrive in a crisis, it's day-to-day living that wears you out. Sometimes I feel like I am trapped in a small recurring drama designed to prove that point. If only there were some way of charging for admission. 'Groundhog Day!' is one of my sister's laments when the same thing happens again and again. But we forget sometimes the message of the movie: not that things repeat themselves, but that within that we can change.

'Bab kashish!' cries Mum from her room.

She has been trying to remember how to say 'shish kebab' for a couple of days now. She has asked me not to tell her, so I don't. It's the kind of mental self-test she likes to run from time to time.

'No,' I say.

'Kiss shabab?'

'No.'

'What's that, then?'

'Nothing. An Islamist rock band. If anything.'

'I don't want any kebab,' says Dad.

'I'm not making any.'

Not for the first time, I am aware that my time here is but a mini-break in a world that has constituted much of my mother's day to day. Nothing like cooking for an unresponsive person to test the limits of who you are. And I must count myself among those hasty and distracted diners at her table. I feel like a celebrity on a television show when they must spend a few hours or days doing something hard or normal. Except I have no other life to scurry back to. This isn't undercover anything. No shortcut to some other, well-paid pantomime. This is it.

In addition to the paper towels deployed around the spills and bellyaches of mealtimes, there's the floating hoard of tissues which must be within arm's reach, wherever we are and at all times. Dad's nose runs constantly, again without diagnosed reason; it is one of the small things which, after a certain age or health-loss milestone, one is supposed to just accept. It gets him down, though, that is, when he is even aware of it. The removal of this moisture is one of my more persistent errands, but a soothing and simple one somehow. It says I'm here and I care, whereas much of what I do say, and I am sure my body language, does not.

Despite this extensive array of available paper, Dad will hoard more tissues in more places than he can keep track of. One advantage of that, if he were the kind of old person prone to, or indeed capable of, wandering off, would be that you could track him by the trail of mansize mishaps that tumble from him like some tragic 2-ply train.

'Box of tissues!' he will cry at any sign I'm heading towards the shops.

'Mogadishu!?' is but one of Mum's many misheard responses, yelled enthusiastically as though in the final round of a quiz, which on some level we are. And if the prize should turn out to be a trip to the war-torn capital of Somalia, I accept it. Gladly. One way.

There are so many tissues lying around that I've developed a kind of snow-blindness. I don't even see them any more. One of the advantages of my sister's less frequent but more frantic visits is that she has an eye for these irregularities and pounces upon them with predatory haste and accompanying cries of outrage. She is the raptor of crap. It doesn't stand a chance against her. She can make the place look better in five minutes than me and the cleaner ever can.

As for toilet paper, I have no idea what they do with it,

except when I know exactly what they do with it. Like the paper towels and tissues, there is constant, often-stated fear of running out. Three rolls visible per toilet seems to be the working minimum.

Add to the paper the food waste: 'Didn't fancy it,' 'Can't risk it,' 'Who bought those anyway?', the Amazon packaging, the fuel, and this house must be worth its weight in Arctic ice each week. And yet, what an economy we are.

In terms of consumption, this is a late-life sprint for the finish. Seldom has so much stuff been consumed by people with so little to do. It occurs to me this might be how the world runs. An unseen grey economy keeping the rest of us busy. Loving serfs in service to a toothless, feudal truth.

13 November 2017

Mum says her pain is worse. I call the doctor. They'll get back to us. Doesn't seem right, her second month of shingles, for things to be deteriorating. What to do?

Dad, as ever, has the best drugs and less need of them, so I swap some of his painkillers for hers. She finds it hard to keep track of what she's taking, though. This indecision and mental fog are new to her. She can't even do the crossword, and this has always been the joy and signal of her agile mind.

I lay pills out at her bedside.

'Those for pain, these for worse pain.'

She doesn't seem to get it and is too sick to pretend otherwise. I say –

'Just call out if it gets bad.'

'What about at night?' she asks.

'OK, let's do it again. These are the strong ones, these come from Dad.'

When she does get up I find her looking at a photo montage of their fiftieth wedding anniversary, ten years ago. It was made by their friend who just died. He assembled it on his computer before he went blind, the faces of each attendee surrounding a picture of my parents.

Mum runs her finger around the circumference of their friends.

'Dead, dead, dead, dead, dead . . .'

This goes on for a while. She is sanguine enough about that but seems disappointed by the picture frame.

'I don't like it,' she announces. 'It looks like something you would get in a shop.'

18 November 2017

My sister comes around with some Complan. Mum hasn't much appetite and this keeps her going. Pink fuel.

We talk about Dad not driving. Should he even try again? My sister, ever one for long-range planning, has put a lot of time into considering how and when our parents should surrender the wheel. Dad's slump in the pub two weeks ago is thus a blessing. He won't fancy it again, she surmises.

I check online. It suggests you should have at least a fortnight off the road if you have fainted. I keep this quiet. Whatever he decides, with Mum as she is, no one is going anywhere fast right now. My sister seems pleased we are car-less. She lost her beloved mother-in-law in a crash. Old people at the wheel is an especially bespoke burden on her ever-restless mind.

I'd settle for restless. All the inner bargaining initially deployed against my situation and the merry mantras of mindfulness have snuffed out through the recent months and left a solid sadness. I feel like someone swapped my guts for a garden gnome. Not just unhappy now, I am afraid. I sense that I am running out of moves. Nothing I know at this point can help me. Maybe no one either. I need something new from someone outside of all this. I call a friend who has had a positive experience in therapy and ask if the person they talk to can recommend someone for me.

Identity Fraud

20 November 2017

I go to London for a day and meet the therapist. Odd, being back in the city where I used to live. I love it but it thrives without me. I am struck by how many adverts there are, and then realize it is not that London has many, but that our hometown has none. It wasn't always the way but it compounds the sense of being forgotten when even capitalism doesn't want you any more. It is a relief just to enter the therapist's building. To have somewhere else to be. Explaining the last year devours most of an hour. Identity, says the therapist, is the essence of this crisis.

'You've left your marriage, lost your job and now you parent your parents.'

Obvious, but I had not seen it laid out so clearly before. This could work. I ask if can come back once a fortnight, she agrees to a discounted fee that makes this feasible. This will be something to do, as well as someone to talk to.

I call the house from the station on the way home, just to see they're all right.

'Who is it?' says Mum.

'Me!'

'Oh. Are you here?'
'No! If I was there I'd be there. I'm here.'
'Oh.'

23 November 2017

I am hoping to walk to Bill's funeral. I must deputize at such things now Mum and Dad are housebound, but my brother pays a visit and, since it's raining, he drives.

This would be unremarkable were it not for his latest choice of vehicle – a lurid sports car that emits a warlike scream at the faintest acceleration. The anti-hearse. Even though he pulls up at the edge of the crematorium, heads turn. A man talks to my brother about fuel consumption as the coffin arrives. I am easily embarrassed, but console myself with the thought that the deceased's background in engineering somehow makes this all right.

Afterwards, the rain has stopped. My brother blasts off and I go for a drink with the family. I see my friend from early childhood for the first time in more than thirty years. He looks the same. I was smart but he was truly, scientifically clever in the mould of his father. He explains to me what he does for a living now and I can sort of grasp it. Then we talk about astronomy and I can't keep up but try not to let this show.

'It's simple,' he says about something which seems complex to me.

I liked that about their house as a kid. They knew things we didn't know. Now his Dad is even further ahead of us.

I walk home wondering when I will next be at the

crematorium. When I get in I realize I have left my raincoat behind, so it turns out to be immediately.

When I get back to the chapel there is no one there, which seems odd as the place is normally a tailback of tears. Each service waiting on the other. But there's nothing. A glitch in mortality, perhaps. Someone eventually lets me in and shows me dozens of dark coats, none of which are mine.

'You said on the phone you had my coat.'

'No,' says the man. 'I said we had black raincoats.'

Must remember to keep an eye out for pedantic obfuscation next time someone round here dies. Equally, if you ever need a black raincoat but lack the budget, now you know where to find them.

*

In the afternoon the practice nurse pays a visit following up the phone call to the surgery. She has brought lidocaine patches for Mum which can be applied directly to where she feels pain. In her case, the red marks that run like bites along her forearm.

The nurse knows my folks.

'Mum seems confused.'

I'd love to argue, but this is undeniable. Instead I shrug.

'I'll come back, take some blood and run the tests on her.'

She means dementia and Alzheimer's, but we don't say as much lest mention of the devil might summon it up.

The patches are immediately effective. Borderline miraculous. So much so I feel angered that we have been at this for months without them. Gratitude is the key, though, and Mum is abundant in that. The absence of pain brings a flurry of movement. She comes downstairs again.

Black Friday

'I've bought a vacuum cleaner.'

Dad has seen an advert in the paper for some cordless article that's a hundred quid less than it could be. That he has (to my knowledge) never used a vacuum cleaner is no obstacle to him picking up the phone and getting one.

'Bloody hell!' says Mum. 'What does he know about cleaning? He's lost his mind.'

What he has lost is a couple of hundred pounds. Enough to merit an intervention. My sister, having a car, will have to take it back. I tell her what's happened over the phone and she is exasperated. I think he was just trying to help. Buying things to make things he doesn't do easier for others is, in its way, kind. Flash new objects in bright boxes have long been code here for 'I love you', even if the buyer never touches what's inside.

Besides, you can't just expect someone to sit in a chair and do nothing, even if that does appear to have been their lifelong aspiration. Buying new stuff is thrilling, I can almost remember the feeling myself. It would be worth setting up a spoof call centre for old people where they can just order things that don't come and are not charged for. Like one of those play shops you have for toddlers, since Dad has mostly forgotten what he has ordered by the time anything arrives.

My sister texts. She is referring to it as 'Dyson-gate'. Everything is a gate now. 'Shit-gate', 'pill-gate', 'biscuit-gate' and so on. If she has designated something 'gate' status and is using a lot of emoticons then I know she has come to terms with it. This is what takes up a lot of your time. Event, respond to event, respond to others' response to event, move on. I have become my parents' PR.

My sister and I discuss the merits of different vacuum cleaners by text.

'Cordless easier to beat someone to death with,' I offer.

'Unless you want to string them up, in which case the flex,' my sister counters.

'Either way,' I respond, 'tidy crime scene.'

Garden Centre of Earthly Delights

27 November 2017

Mum is talking about going outside. She still seems a little out of her mind, but I am not about to say no to a ride.

She has set her sights on the garden centre.

'I want Christmas cards,' she declares. 'Coconut halves to hang up for the birds.'

I can't recall the last time she even talked about the future. She takes an hour and a half to get ready.

There has been no public appearance for a month or more and the make-up and clothes that might ordinarily have been in pole position must be found, selected and applied. Last time she stepped out it was a different season. And so this simple trip assumes the status of a state occasion. But before we can call a taxi we must consider those we leave behind.

Dad's anxiety about being alone will fall and rise. The last time he got antsy and we all thought he was paranoid, it turned out to be an impending heart attack. The same heart attack that brought me home back in February. The point and the problem being that aimless anxiety and justified panic look the same from the outside.

Garden Centre of Earthly Delights

Since that admission, which also raised the spectre of Mum alone in the house when Dad is hospitalized, we have taken what we deem to be appropriate measures. Chief among these is an 'alert-call' system: an emergency button worn about the old person's person, which, when pressed, signals a call centre who then contact the house through a dedicated microphone and speaker unit and ask if they're all right. If the caller is too unwell to answer or too far away, the call centre agents contact the emergency services. This costs just a few pounds a month and seems an excellent innovation. Yet nothing here is straightforward.

To set up the system I had to check its range and figured that the furthest my parents could ever go without leaving altogether would be the far end of the garden. I made my way to the back fence to run a test but was overwhelmed by memory instead. It was up here, behind a tree since felled, that I hid, sometime in the 1970s, having packed a bag and announced I was leaving home. I waited for a search party that was never sent and went back in when I got hungry, like generations of melodramatic children before and since. This was forty years ago. I had better odds of escape at eight years old.

Nine months after I set up the call system, Dad, characteristically, will not be separated from his alert button. He keeps it like a talisman although he struggles to remember how it works. If I ask him to test it, he talks into the button, asking it for help as if it were a telephone. Mum forgets to wear hers and when she does, accidentally activates it. She has a 'trick' for opening tin cans (all packaging becomes a maddening struggle for the elderly finger), using a wooden spoon to lever up the ring pull. The spoon catches the button and sounds the alert, which she won't necessarily be able to hear the response to. She then shuffles about the kitchen hunting for the source of the alarm while Dad attempts to direct her by yelling from another room, like a cruel reimagining of *The Crystal Maze*. Somehow this, ostensibly a safety mechanism, has yet to yield an unnecessary ambulance or cause an injury that requires one.

As Operation Garden Centre approaches, I run pre-flight checks with my father. Alert-call button, landline, mobile phone, inhalers, angina spray and tissue after tissue and biscuits all in reach of his chair. His empire at his elbow.

'We will be back within an hour.'

He shrugs slightly, which I interpret as 'anything could happen'. I have in the past deployed the phrase, 'If you need round-the-clock care . . .' in these moments, implying institutionalization to forestall accusations of abandonment, but we don't come to that today.

The balance between his anxiety and our mother's freedom from it is one of the tougher judgements of their care, perhaps even their relationship. Quite what these two get from one another, beyond the basic caveman metrics of the shelter-for-services deal, can be hard to see sometimes, but there is something more than mere proximity here. A love that's no one else's business.

Whatever reassurance he derives from knowing an eighty-nine-year-old deaf woman is asleep upstairs, it is real to him. Now she is risen, he will worry when she is not there. There is comfort in knowing you are not alone, even if your companion could nap through a nuclear war.

'You have my mobile number.' I hold out the cell phone for added clarity.

He frowns warily, looking past the phone towards the end of the garden. As though some enemy might be gathered just inside the tree line, waiting for the old lady to go out before descending to claim ships' barometers, broken radios, Lowry prints and the other ephemera of their lives. I'm not saying there are not bad things out there. I just don't think we are the kind of target over which disaster has to bide its time.

I call a cab and guide Mum down the steps. She's thrilled just to take the air. The garden centre is new to me and she guides me around it, her arm in mine. It is painfully slow and yet a strange kind of pleasure. To be leaned on and not to yield. What more can we do?

It is an old crowd in here, but Mum might be the eldest. People who are merely in their seventies or early eighties clutch their plants and let us pass. As with dogs or infants, folk are far nicer to you when you've someone this old along for the ride. It raises my faith in the species. Even myself. By the time we reach the till I feel pride.

Mum poses outside; unaided, smiling and victorious. I take a picture and send it to my siblings. It is a campaign image, though. Propaganda. She is exhausted as soon as we are back. The pain returns. The relief from the patches is purely symptomatic and they are strictly rationed. I see online that the residual nerve pain, neuralgia, from shingles can last years, a lifetime in some cases. Whatever that might mean within these walls is hard to gauge, but I say nothing.

Mum returns to bed. Talk of the future is replaced by fretful and familiar questions about sleeping pills and pain relief. I bring drugs and mugs of soup. I hang the coconut halves out for the birds, but when I open the curtains so she can watch she is too weak to sit up and asks they be closed again. Bar the usual wobble to the bathroom that will be it for her tonight. All things considered, this is a very good day.

All Things Must Pass

28 November 2017

My sister drops ready meals to the house, and with drugs and drudgery taken care of I head to London, looking for life and work and sanity. Nothing cooking. When I get back here there have been serious amendments to the kitchen.

After thirty years, the last of which have required a mix of wilful blindness and innovation to go on, the cooker here has had it. Its greasy dials dive lemming-like from its stained face towards the nearby bin. Each failing aspect of, or appliance in the house is fraught with memory and metaphor, but the time comes when you must put something out of its misery and move on. Now a sleek black glass replacement squats modishly in its faulty predecessor's place, making the house look Neolithic by comparison. Its clock is all zeroes, blinking for my attention while Mum squints suspiciously from across the room.

I know the squint is a matter of mood rather than a vision thing as Dad has, in typical style, seized upon a mooted suggestion and hired someone to massively overreact to it. In this case, the kitchen lighting. The boudoir twilight which has for years enfolded the business end of their kitchen has been augmented now by a blinding LED better suited to dental surgery, prison courtyards or deliberate sleep deprivation.

'It's like a bloody takeaway,' says Mum, who, despite being partial to outbreaks of deep-fried cholesterol, has no wish to feel 'like I work in a fish and chip shop'.

The domestic grime enabled by the macular degeneration of my folks (and my eyes aren't getting any sharper) is much discussed. There are times when it is tough to mask your exasperation as you reach for something clean and realize that what you're holding is dirty. Mugs of old Horlicks, hard as cement. Forgotten cups of milk in the microwave. Lost continents of crumbs. I'm not even sure this newly acquired second sun will help. But Dad has arranged something, and that is not nothing. As the shortest day approaches, he has bought illumination.

That night, a ferocious storm. The house rattles and the rains whip at it. Safe inside, it feels good to have some context, to feel oneself upon a wilder planet, instead of hearing nothing but our own frail sounds.

Timber Land

29 November 2017

A tall tree from the house behind us has been torn up in the gale and now sprawls across the garden. Tree surgeons are already upon it with chainsaws. I throw a coat over the age-slackened tracksuit that has become my default uniform. I was quite a fussy dresser, once, if I thought I might bump into anyone, though something of a slob at home. This tendency has spread now and metastasized. If something foul happens here it tends to do so in the morning; I have learnt not to bother showering or 'properly' dressing till midday. In yesterday's clothes I duck outside.

When I was a kid I thought all jobs looked interesting. As an out-of-work adult I'm the same. Worse, even. Childhood and unemployment have the same feeling for me: I just want to join in with something. The tree surgeons are skilled, amiable, thriving as a team. They have cool neon outerwear and shining climbing equipment. Unadorned as they appear to be by ancient sportswear, catheter leakage, poor life choices and porridge stains, I am free to project onto and idealize their lives, about which I know nothing, until I have topped up my own sadness to the required level. I don't do much social media and so am reliant on the real world for a fix of this kind of self-curated pain.

Dad has long been engaged in a Canute-style showdown against nature in the form of an oak tree outside. On late midsummer afternoons the full foliage of the oak casts a section of his patio into shade and he has for years now sought to have the tree trimmed or taken down.

From my bed I can see the oak's upper branches and have since childhood marked the seasons through its changes. Over the decades I have hidden behind it, pissed against it, failed to climb it and accidentally almost burned it to the ground. Nowadays it stands as a point of scale and reference, a sign that there are older shapes and systems and lives beyond our own. If the Old Man wants to do something I am, in all respects except the physical, powerless against him. Not short of things to get angry about or anger to assign, I am afraid of how it might feel if I were to come back one day and find the oak, this living landmark, maimed or downed.

Happily, the tree has a local protection order on it. Thwarted by the council in his attempts at deforestation, Dad has done what he will do in any situation that displeases or challenges him – offered likely-looking men cash to solve it on his behalf. No questions asked. All reputable tree surgeons are thus aware of him.

'Is he in there still?' asks this one, nodding toward the house. Indeed.

'Surprised he's still alive,' he adds, not unkindly.

Still alive and still, like Ahab, planning how to oust the tree that torments his ailing frame, as it waves at him through the window. He is too weak now to go outside and rage against its shade. If he lives to see another summer, all this will replay again.

It is sad how little interest any of this outdoor drama evokes inside. Mum would have been down the garden with cups of tea not so long ago. Now she's back in bed again, waiting for the new drugs to take hold. I look for the flicker of pirate gold in the Old Man's eyes when I tell him there are men with chainsaws here, but he doesn't seem bothered. How times change.

Deliverance

The days themselves are short, dark shocks. The light apologetic. Needed elsewhere. In a profound temporal reversal I feel as though time moves so slowly here that we have become science fiction, the crew of a lone spaceship. Suspended animation, sleeping mostly. Heading further from the sun. Nothing really happens, but it takes so long.

My friend Dave drives me to London, and we do what our generation do instead of writing Christmas cards to one another. We stand in a huge room and listen to a band play loud music we used to take drugs and dance to. It helps. I am glad that I can still get someone on the guest list for something, I have some residual agency there. But being driven back down the empty motorway I feel childlike again. And not in a good way. I lost my grip on the wheel of fortune, then it reversed over me.

3 December 2017

With nothing left of last night but tinnitus and a backstage pass, I cut the lidocaine patches and stick them to Mum's body.

Each day she does a little more. As she reclaims her terrain she obsesses about running out of pain relief.

'The patches?' she asks.

'Plenty.'

'What day is it?'

She wants to know in case the chemist and the doctor are closed.

'Don't worry about it,' I reply, since I have no idea what day it is either any more.

★

We stumble across drugs here without trying. If I open a cupboard or a drawer or even an envelope in the spirit of inquiry as to what might have remained in the decades since I left home, the answer, mostly, is that whatever I remembered has vanished and been replaced by drugs.

You might question what it matters, that a forty-eight-year-old man wondering if his bath toys had survived, instead finds a drawer filled with out-of-date Senokot. Yet somehow it does. The costs to the NHS, the cursed ubiquity of it all, the temptation to swallow something just for the ride. It plays on my mind.

5 December 2017

Conscience gets the better of me, and I finally look our drug problem in the eye, quantifying what we have in every room and cupboard. As though finally lifting a long-picked scab, I am appalled but also fascinated by what's discovered. The truth is we live in a kind of prescription stash house. The amount of drugs here is insane.

The root of the surplus is my father. Much of Dad's pharmaceutical mountain and the surrounding dunes of drugs date from before he was *really* ill, as though he were prepping for this eventuality. And yet his every step further into the arena of the unwell is matched by a new delivery from the chemist. None of the old stuff was ever finished because new stuff is always on its way. I am on first-name terms with the pharmacists in town and greet their couriers like old friends as they trot up the steps.

When I initially realized my parents got medication delivered for free I thought this was excellent. But the old man's paranoia runs as deep as his memory doesn't. He will reorder what I order and then order more again. It's like the hypochondriac's Deliveroo.

The old drugs cannot be recycled and my father's ability to generate, sustain and contract fresh ailments and conditions is an act of such sustained creativity that in any other walk of life but dying his work would be in a museum. I take it upon myself (like I have much else to do) to make a change.

There is a kind of silence the Old Man can generate which has become far more powerful than an outright 'no', and it is this that meets me if I ask if we can throw 'this' out. 'This' can be anything. Even an old tissue plucked from the trail.

'We don't need this, do we?' I will ask, holding a Kleenex at arm's length.

He shrugs. Better old tissues than no tissues. Better this than an answer.

In the case of the drugs his silence is especially forthright. So I just stop asking.

Deliverance

Out they go: antibiotics, analgesics, anticoagulants; these are just the tip of the alphabet. For a while I google things to see if they are noteworthy, fatal or fun. Nothing is. So it goes in the bin or back to the chemist, or to my sister's friend who runs an underground railroad for medicine to more desperate countries, till all we have is all we are presently prescribed.

There is a moment of something like relief when it appears to be over. But I am nagged by a powerful sense that I have missed something, that there must be more. Fans of seventies movies will recall Gene Hackman's Popeye Doyle experiencing a similar sensation with a car he thinks is full of heroin in *The French Connection.*

And if there's one terrible lesson we can learn from movies, it's that our instincts are never wrong. Thus I am guided by the spirit of Popeye to my father's wardrobe, and there it is, pharma-Narnia. Temazepam Aslan squats at the back, behind a veil of blazers – a micro-motherlode of prescription pharmaceuticals that could keep an Irvine Welsh character occupied for months.

Yet this feels like a transgression. This is, after all, his private stash. I am only acting on the discomfort of myself and others about the drugs we knew of. And so like the good-ish son and first-rate schemer I am, I take a blister pack of pristine tranquillizers and call it a day. He can have the rest. There is a bottle of Bacardi hidden here as well. He doesn't drink Bacardi. Then it dawns on me: the Old Man might have a plan.

Into the Valet

Walking back down the hill, I notice the car is now on the drive. How could that have happened? The answer, as with most vehicular surprises in our lives, is my brother. He has chaperoned Dad on a local trip and now deems him fit to be back on the road.

This is very much my brother's MO. Appear suddenly, act decisively. There are instances when this feels like divine intervention, and other times when the disregard for my awareness of the day-to-day minutiae of this situation feels like a twist of the knife. This would be in the latter category.

When a family is reassembled, as we are, for one last job, few things go to plan. As in some misguided heist movie, there is much haggling over methods, collisions of motives and spiralling subplots, all complicated by the decay of any previous hierarchy. Newton's third law gets amplified when everything must be repeated several times. Every action has endless reactions. No one is really in charge. Sometimes I think I am the boss, sometimes just the narrator. When it comes to the driving argument I tend to step aside.

Into the Valet

Growing up, my brother had posters of vehicles on his wall, and from scooter to sports car has always been astride an engine. I fell in love with and then stalled at pushbikes, and that was that. That Dad is willing to drive again, to leave the chair and dream of life beyond the front door, is excellent. But is it wise? My brother believes so. The neural processes deployed, he contends, are less likely to wither.

'What else is he gonna do?'

This makes a certain sense, but I am as anxious about the cost of any highway carnage on strangers as I am about marginal gains in the old boy's cortex.

Dad is musing about where to drive tomorrow, then asks –

'What's for dinner?'

I send a text update to my sister about Dad driving, which I know will precipitate a discourse that will rival the Warren Commission. I put some lamb chops under the grill and prepare for a long night.

The chops are a strategic choice. My gambit is that their scent might draw my mother from upstairs. I don't eat meat. Fish has become a common compromise here in order to avoid cooking multiple meals too often. But if you really want a reaction, to see pleasure and anticipation in your diners' eyes at this table, then something with hooves will have to die. The politics and personal choices of my abstinence are neither here nor there in this context. I see my parents' meals as an extended death-row dinner. They can have more or less what they like.

I like cooking. One of the few times in life you can say with any certainty that you are not wasting your time. This pays double when Mum takes the bait and joins us downstairs. She does, however, undercut this small success by announcing that she isn't enjoying food.

'I've no appetite,' she says, between mouthfuls.

After a brief but silent wave of resentment I must reflect that she is not given to mean-spirited assessments or a plodding attitude, even in late life. To see her eat mechanically is testament to how weak she has become. I steer them to the living room for *Coronation Street*, crank up Radio 3 in the kitchen and set about the pots to the sound of German opera. In an act of either tribute or defiance the dishwasher here stopped working properly when Margaret Thatcher died.

7 *December 2017*

We are back in the car for the first time in over a month. Testament to Dad's love of his vehicle is that the places he wants to drive to are for the benefit of the car. In 'plenty of reassurance but zero expertise' mode as usual, I sit beside him as we head up to the garage. I fill her up and pay, a chance to see my smiling friend behind the counter. Next Dad wants it cleaned and drives us into town, to a place I've never been before, a manual car wash that has sprung up by where the football ground once stood. You stay inside the vehicle while people wash and shine the bodywork. We share a moment as the work goes on outside.

'Been coming here a few years now,' he says, 'they do a good job.'

There is something in this which reminds me again this is a human being with their own rituals and routines as opposed to just a bump in my road, which is how it feels sometimes. I am grateful to my brother's initiative for this moment of mostly silent paternal bonding. If we plough into someone now, it will all have been worthwhile.

Shelf Life

8 December 2017

'I need a new book,' announces Mum.

Dad is too short of breath to drive today and so, after the usual prolonged preparations, Mum and I are on our way in a taxi to the library. She taught me to read here. She knows the building well but now can't recall the layout, and staggers about purposefully having wrestled free from my arm.

It is painful, twilight-of-a-champion stuff to watch her attempt to navigate the shelves. A librarian approaches and asks her what she'd like. She yells back –

'NOTHING TOO PROFOUND!'

Our everyday volume brings the place to a standstill, not that much was happening to begin with. The librarian steers her to where superficiality abounds.

I find the health and well-being section and search for something that might speak to our predicament. But other life stages, birth and bereavement, claim the shelves here. Meanwhile Mum reappears, laden with historical and spy fiction. I try and scan these using the digital system they've installed, but fail. I am about to ask for help when, in a stark reminder that neither progress nor decline is ever linear, she takes the books and scans them herself.

This moment of apparent victory is short-lived. When we get home she looks at the pile of books.

'I'm not sure what I've got these for.'

I'm out at the shops when the practice nurse comes but get back as she is leaving. Mum, she says, has passed her MMSE or mini-mental state examination 'with flying colours'. This is joyous news. Mum says nothing but stomps about with something like triumph, then goes back to bed. As promised, the nurse has taken blood for further testing.

Despite the positive assessment it remains essential to bear witness to these things since information retention is next to non-existent here. Who comes to the house, whether they came, and what it might have meant are low on the menu of memories, and in ever smaller print. I have become a cynical detective. If I didn't see it I can't be sure it happened, and I do need this case closed.

PART TWO

Nowhere Plans

In one of the many operational hypocrisies that make up our days, while I steal and consume drugs from my father, I would prefer it if Mum didn't do the same. Now up and about, she's testifying to the mental stresses she has suffered in her prone state. It's been two months since shingles first laid her low.

'I can't tell you what I think about at night,' she says, with a sadness so uncharacteristic that I am determined to do something about it right away. Something holistic or natural perhaps?

'And I have a . . . woman's problem.'

She nods sadly towards her thighs. That remains beyond my jurisdiction and ideally will remain so. The organic approach can wait. I make her a doctor's appointment.

Confident the car looks peerless, Dad, breathing freely this morning, turns his attention to his own appearance and decides he needs a trim. His hair has been the same since 1973, as far as I can see. Likewise, I myself am stuck mentally somewhere around the age of fifteen. The rest is detail. Dad's hair getting too long would constitute a major upheaval, a rip in the fabric of our space and time. Best get this done.

Ever keen to push herself, Mum wants to come for the ride. And so we get the gang together. Dad takes the wheel; Mum sits behind us.

Like us our city's centre is no longer as it was. An eviscerated high street, heavy traffic, parking distant from the shops . . . all this and more have shifted my folks' retail affections to an old town up the road where my dad has his hair cut since his previous barber died.

Mum is uncharacteristically silent and pensive on the ride and doesn't leave the car while Dad has his trim, so I wait with her once I've helped him inside. When he's done he plays the blue badge card and parks on the high street while I run into the chemist and get herbal sleeping aids and chamomile tea for Mum. The queue in there is long, each customer attended with fresh levels of ineptitude and inertia, so that I wonder if there is a way to freebase chamomile to keep me calm.

They are sitting in the car, oblivious to the considerable tailback behind them. I'm halfway in when Dad says –

'Can you get me some gloves?'

I am about to ask him why he would need any, given that he doesn't go out, when I realize that our location disproves that premise, although the car is so hot you wouldn't risk leaving a dog in it. Dad is pointing towards the somehow still thriving department store across the road. Avoiding eye contact with the traffic building up around us I cut across the street and run inside.

No wonder they like it here. The shop is playing by the rules of another century and has the clientele to prove it. The staff, too. In the e-commerce era, this is where retail comes to die in its lover's arms. A hospice of habit. A cultural retirement home.

In a curious but forlorn attempt to seem modern, the menswear department is adorned by a large cardboard figure of Jim Morrison. Jim Callaghan would be more on the money. They do not appear to be selling leather pants, LSD or any of the Lizard King's signature items. I can only conclude then that he is placed here by the Fates to further torment me. I was a teenage Doors fan, and so the singer's presence as I queue for gloves amongst the dying becomes another rebuke. He died young in the bath from an overdose. I missed that bus, and not for want of trying. I miss the bath too. All we have now is a walk-in shower and what's left of our pride. Even in this place, in mid-morning and mid-life, I suddenly feel old and tired. I grab myself some gloves for good measure. The Old Man is onto something. It is cold outside.

I return to the car and am about to get in and release the arterial blockage we have caused to the town when I remember I am also supposed to pick up a diary. That Mum has even asked for a space to map out another year is heartening; I am not about to let her down. I pelt into the newsagent and find one in the all-important week-on-a-page format my parents prefer. People in cars are so angry by now that I shield my face from them behind the diary like a suspect coming out of court.

'Drive!' I say to Dad, and like the world's oldest accomplice he gently puts his foot down.

★

Halfway around the one-way system that should take us home Dad asks –

'Have you seen the horse?' I have no idea what this means.

Then he reminds me. There is a new statue in the park here commemorating equine service in the Great War. I know better than to question acts of martial memorializing in front of this crowd; besides, he has turned off for it already.

In a life made more of flashbacks than forward motion I am propelled into the past again. Reminded of those drives as a kid when I needed to pee and found my pleas unheeded. Sitting in the front does nothing to reduce the vestigial sense of abduction as we drive. At least when I was young we had bladders in common. We would have to stop eventually. Now Dad is catheterized, this need never end.

When we reach the park it's raining and neither of them will leave the car. Instead I am dispatched alone to admire the sculpture. I trudge the river path to where I'm told it stands. The operational sadness within me is infused with a wave of such glutinous remorse that I feel as if I might fall over.

Remorse for everything. For the condition of being alive. I can taste it on my teeth like metal, the bitterness of knowing there is no one else to blame. All I can see are happier times and the impossibility of their recovery. My child self, darting about this same path. My adult self, recalling my wife when once we walked here, back when we were young and happy. Then this. Self-made loneliness and more and death to follow. Pinned between losses, that which I have left and those who will be taken.

Now I see it. A sculpted metal horse, life-sized. Ragged as the bandaged bronze soldier that holds its reins. Their heads bowed. How do you bring your own small sadness to the sum of grief that this alludes to? But between the glorious dead and the still just-living in the car behind me, it strikes me (and maybe this is the mission of memorials) there is space to do something. This is not a movie. There are no rewinds, rewrites, or director's cuts. Pull yourself together.

I head back to the car, wipe the tears and rain from my face and get inside, not caring for the moment where we go or how we get there.

Obligation to Participate

10 December 2017

We describe Mum's mood and sleeping issues to the doctor, who says the blood tests have confirmed her non-dementia diagnosis. She prescribes mirtazapine, 'used in depression complicated by anxiety or trouble sleeping', apparently. Sounds about right. It might take a month to work, the doctor says. Mum must persist with it. That we can live with. Persistence is what we do.

Mum does her best to get back to some kind of normal. I return from errands and the odd psychotherapeutic flit to London and too often find this means her doing remedial tasks for the Old Man.

He simply has, by virtue of his life at sea, little idea of how to look after himself and, I think, no ready model of the reciprocal, signified warmth that might fuel a happier home. As a defector from a marriage of my own I am doubly sensitive to accusations of male ineptitude. I have my issues, no doubt and no wonder. But on the domestic front Dad is sometimes at the back of a class of his own.

I do my best to defend him. My sister is keeper of some

heartfelt, tidal judgement which ebbs and flows; my mother more sniper-like in her outbreaks of disdain. But there is an artful streak I recognize too well about my father's being that makes this harder. Add that to the invisible inner Jenga of this whole situation, and the seemingly simple request: tissue, biscuit, remote control . . . can cause the leaning tower of one's tolerance to collapse.

'You want a tea?' I'll ask.

'No, I'm all right,' he'll say.

Next thing I know Mum is shambling towards him with a brew in her hand.

'I just asked you if you wanted a tea!'

'I didn't want one then.'

'Ask me if I'm here. Not her.'

'I couldn't see you.'

'What are you saying?' asks Mum and I prise the mug from her hand and hand it to him.

'The tea's for Dad.'

'I KNOW WHO IT'S FOR!'

'Don't shout.'

To see her buckling beneath the latest non-essential request like some Brueghel peasant in a painting is a ready source of resentment. However defensive and unprepared I am about the oak tree and what might befall it, is nothing to how I feel about my mother.

I once asked my dad for advice on a serious matter and he said, with great assurance –

'Sometimes there's nothing you can do.'

I'm guessing the early loss of his own mother hardwired

this into his world view. Which is not to say he's wrong, just that I can't quite find that level of acceptance myself. Especially when it comes to Mum and Dad. Especially when his needs step up, stagger and threaten to collapse into hers.

As I boil the kettle again a bird thuds into the window. A wagtail, male, I presume, which rises regularly from the bushes to attack its own reflection. Part of what I am tasked with is to make sure that my mother doesn't destroy herself simply through her own conditioning, striving against the equally blameless glass of my father's expectation. We are creatures of deep routine here. Us and the bird. At least the bird has certainty. I look at next year's empty diary and consider my next move.

11 *December 2017*

The rise and fall of one's moods and the subtle vibrations of hypervigilance add to the fact that being here is physically tiring. Heat, work and worry combine. This is one of those days when I feel empty, as if there were an open spigot to my soul. You leak out into the carpet, like the radiator in Dad's room. There is something to our predicament that takes a spiritual toll.

By way of respite I ride to my friend Dave's house. A ten-minute cycle, stretches of which you can complete no-handed if large parts of you are still somehow thirteen years old. He and I have been close since we were actually thirteen. He commutes to London and, like one of his kids, some evenings I find myself waiting for him to get home. The relief of talking things over with someone who knows me this well, but with whom I share no DNA, is incalculable. It is confession, in a sense. Also his house has actual young people in it and isn't as hot as a pizza oven. There and elsewhere I drink, complain and make light of it all. Sometimes a truth slinks out.

'It sounds like looking after children,' says Dave's partner. This is a kind and intuitive cliché, to which I have a darkly polished answer:

'If you wish your children sudden, painless deaths each time you say goodnight and leave their rooms . . .'

This is the fact of it. Dad first, and soon, ideally. If only for practical reasons. Mum could get by without him, up to a point; the reverse is impossible. The longer this lasts, the worse it will be and perhaps the worse I will become. The more of us there are, the faster we sink. Our life is a leaking lifeboat. Or so it seems to me.

In psychology and ethics this is known as a Trolley Problem, after a model in which one might change the direction of a runaway tram to spare one group of people, but in doing so kill another. There is no 'right' answer, but as Wikipedia explains, 'Under some interpretations of moral obligation, simply being present in this situation and being able to influence its outcome constitutes an obligation to participate.' My mind plays like a *Hamlet* prequel. No ghosts or murders, yet. Everyone's alive, but not for long.

'You do the best you can,' I confess. 'But you can't help wishing it was over.'

Dave's kitchen falls silent, not with shock but recognition. Even those who have not faced it expect to feel the same.

Hugged and heard, I ride home on all the guilt and conflict that such a troubled love evokes. My hands stay on the handle-bars. It is all uphill in this direction.

My sister texts:

'Any thoughts re Christmas presents?'

'Dignitas voucher.'

'Who for?!'

Bags of Life

Feeling somehow far from home while also stuck inside it, there is no way out this morning as it is grocery delivery day.

My sister has sanctioned Mum from heavy shopping, but this does not stop the Old Lady from trying to get to the supermarket and doing it anyway. My sister (to whom I am quite content to assign the harsher role) begs and then nags her about using a walking stick.

'Those are for old people,' is Mum's retort as she wobbles away to the shops.

'If she falls . . .' My sister has begun this sentence so often that there is no reason to end it, not that that will stop her.

'Broken hip, dementia, death!' is one of her most beloved pessimistic chants.

As ever, amid the stream of dark truisms, she has a point. It is difficult. You can't just tie them to a chair, apparently.

Against this dissonance the online grocery shop has fallen to that renowned specialist in e-commerce, my father. He jabs madly at his tablet in this strange and expensive version of bingo. We wait and see what turns up. He and Mum have some inbuilt resistance – based on years of practice – to discussing what they actually need or want. She makes lists and doesn't show them to him. He orders things without asking her, then forgets what he has bought and buys it again. Born and raised above a shop, he now does all he can to keep them going.

What transpires is madness. Costly, chaotic and wasteful. But one of the fascinating and perhaps liberating aspects of this life is when you come face to face with your limitations. For all the things I can do, going through the online grocery shop with Dad is just too much. I would rather do the physical stuff. Somehow the border of the ancient and modern on which the grocery order balances is just too hot a beat for me. I can't handle it. I have to walk away lest I run screaming over the horizon. The final straw is everywhere, sometimes.

Some father-son relationships are founded on shared experiences of getting things done. Fixing cars, perhaps, untangling fishing lines. I have none of these memories, despite being raised in the heyday of killing fish for kicks and leaded petrol. Like later generations, me and the Old Man have swapped the roar of engines for the taps, clicks and silences of the online age. Only the outbursts of profanity remain the same. If you want to see how much you love someone, try and fix their computer.

'Password?'

'Don't know.'

'User ID?'

'Don't know.'

I would consider taking my own life and the lives of others before dealing with the online 'help' desk of his email provider again, bearing so little basic information. No Trolley Problems there. If anything gets logged out of now that will be end of his online adventures.

★

Into this stable instability land the groceries. A spin-off of the Amazon issue, except this is about things we need. If I am not there to monitor the delivery, one or both of two things will happen.

Either my mother will struggle to unpack it and give my dad a hard time about all the things he has or hasn't ordered and the expense of all this, or my sister will arrive and unpack it herself along with a diatribe against the whole household, which she will save and relay to me another time. To avoid the endless repetition of such feelings I try to intercept all the food and booze and tissues and whatever else is coming before it's halfway up the drive.

Food is an arena in which I have observed and absorbed one of the fundamental laws of elderly supervision:

Dysfunction *is* function.

Getting things wrong or confused is how they get by. If one can accept that, as I have in this particular realm, then things are simpler. If you take arms against it, as my sister seems to, then your better nature can perish in the fight, and God knows I have little enough of that to go around.

This is one of the great dangers of 'care'. It can consume us so that it will mask and even perjure the love it might be founded on. If you are not careful you live all your time in crisis mode. Adrenaline claims you, and too soon that feels normal. Also, much of this is just the modern world. Nothing personal. Digital dislocation abounds.

So I don't mind the unpacking. There are no fruit or vegetables sometimes, but chocolates, shellfish and a bottle of good malt whisky instead. We work round it. I can pick up the rest, as could Mum, pre-shingles. Money is wasted but thank God there is money to waste. It is over the actual waste that I will lose my rag.

It is not so much the packaging as the meat. I accept that since I don't eat the stuff I have a bias, but the animals slain, bought and then thrown out here could populate the ark, albeit an ark made mostly of ham, tongue and bacon.

'Dad likes a tongue sandwich,' says Mum defensively, as I question why, again, I am throwing great outdated slabs of it away.

She is oblivious to the built-in innuendo of this hateful snack. Others are not. If she mentions Dad's preference in front of my brother, a lifelong *Viz* subscriber, he can't contain himself. The implied imagery prevents me from sharing his amusement. Somewhat inconsistently, I struggle when Mum refers to the radiator in the Old Man's bedroom as 'Dad's pipe'.

Raised in the Depression and then under rationing, my parents are making up for it now. Perhaps they see this as a kind of extended after-show-party-cum-trolley-dash, where they can eat what they want, however ridiculous, since the main event is over. When the unpacking is done the kitchen table now looks less like the centre of a family home than a touring rock band's backstage rider. Except we have more drugs, and better whisky.

Malt Risky

13 December 2017

Alcohol amid the meat and medicines has become a concern. As a family we are not untouched by addiction, far from it, but this has not been an issue for my folks themselves. Until now. Dad's persistent purchase of Scotch has become a trigger for anxieties and a certain sublimated rage among the women in our group who do the most to serve him. And, to a growing extent, me too. Especially given that, over and above more dramatic ailments, his most presenting and painful condition, lately, is gout.

Unlike the cancers, the heart problems, the kidneys, the general oldness, but somewhat like the COPD and the diabetes, there is a certain reading of events here in which getting gout is the Old Man's fault. Summoning whisky, wine and marine invertebrates to the house when the condition means others have to serve them to you, is like blowing smoke in the face of someone helping you with lung cancer and asking them to light you another. He did at least abandon cigarettes in his seventies. Dad's drinking, then, on the one hand a charismatic rebuke to his circumstances, is also decried. Dad's latest bottle looks beguiling. Even the LED chip shop light refracts through the golden liquid like a sign from heaven. A summons. When the dinner things are put away I break the seal, sit at the kitchen table, take a drink and consider its costs.

Over the years, uric acid deposits in the joints of gout sufferers and crystallizes. These accumulations are known as tophi. In Dad's case they present as spare satanic toes that have sprouted and spread on all sides of his feet like knuckles of root ginger.

'Have you seen Dad's feet?' my brother asked me a few years back.

I nodded in the manner of one asked by a fellow soldier if he had served in some disastrous battle. For years Dad dismissed them as bunions, then the truth emerged in hospital this summer. Or rather, the bunion myth collapsed and made carnage of my father's credibility from which it may never fully emerge.

I was at his bedside when the rheumatologists came. Both doctors paled as they pulled back the sheets.

After a moment's silence the consultant surveyed his junior, who could only shrug, shake his head and swallow. I felt, for a second, oddly proud.

When the men had recovered, the consultant delivered his verdict.

'Tophi,' a hint of wonder in his voice, implying, 'but not as we know it.' 'Gouty tophi,' he added out loud.

'No sensation?'

The Old Man shook his head.

'We should maybe . . .' stammered the underling.

'Get the others,' confirmed the consultant.

The junior photographed my father's feet from several angles.

'Fame at last,' I said.

I don't remember if Dad laughed. I hope so, since a storm was duly coming. The doctors left, their morning doubtless made.

I can understand Dad's inner bargain, since I have the same instinct for self-deception. 'Eat what you want, and you'll die before it matters' will have been the headline here. I have for years defended him against my mum and sister's accusations that he is wilfully more decrepit than necessary, occasionally backed by documentary evidence – diabetes diet sheets and leaflets of grim warnings stuffed down the side of sofas and so on – so I am to some degree complicit in the cover-up.

Earlier this year, before the rheumatologist's reveal, when Dad appeared to be dying and we had held hands in hospital, said goodbye and been through all that together, my brother and I would take Scotch to his ward in a plastic bottle. The look on his face when he tasted it after weeks of confinement and distress was among the happiest I have seen him. The doctors and nurses weren't bothered. The consultant, openly astonished at the Old Man's survival, said it would be fine. Then Dad recovered and came home. 'Came', though, suggests some agency on his behalf. You go and collect them, like an item repaired.

It is one thing to raise whisky to another's lips in hospital where the state will catch and clean the outcomes. Quite another, when it is one of multiple requests, framed as demands, that must be met at home. In the months of survival since I moved back in and his last long hospitalization, I have cultivated a compromise around the Scotch. For a few weeks it was one for him and one for me. But like strange athletes, one must coach and coax the aged back into the everyday via careful motivation. So I decided – you are well enough for whisky when you can get up and pour it for yourself, but I will stand beside you all the way as we try.

Scotch, then, became the amber carrot which lured the Old Man from his chair.

'You can do it,' I would say to him, and up he would rise.

First on his frame, then just a stick. Miracles happen. Unassisted he now stands nightly, circa 17.30, makes his way slowly to the kitchen and fetches himself a malt. More than a finger, a deeper measure, anointed with a shot of water.

It was like this that the reviled habit became a signifier of health. First it was the Scotch, then he was back at the kettle. Next, a self-made sandwich. Which is as good as it has ever got.

Yet the bottle remains a rebuke. The 'clank' as it hits the kitchen tile when he is done transcends my mother's deafness and tweaks some aged irritation in her soul. If she goes out to the recycling (another errand which it is impossible to deflect her from entirely) she returns grumbling about the empties.

There is more afoot here than anyone can fix, although the mind goads us to try. Physical health, mental health, the specifics of an ancient union, you can drive yourself mad trying to manage all this stuff. Their stuff. On this basis, then, I allow myself to allow the drinking and, when possible, intercept the consternation around it. If I am missing something here, then it must stay lost for now.

I pour myself another. Mum trundles back into the kitchen and notices the blind is open. A faux pas. She reaches over and wrestles with the cord.

'I'll pull this down,' she announces. 'So people can't see all the fun we're having.'

Kitchens of Distinction

14 December 2017

Mum says the mirtazapine isn't making any difference. I have told her to wait, like I know what I'm talking about. Meantime she makes forays into domesticity, attempting to reclaim the kitchen, to reassert herself. I won't stand in her way here, quite the reverse.

If she can cook a simple meal again then I am liberated. I don't know what I would do with the time this might buy me, but right now, just the possibility of an interlude is enough. This morning she starts chopping vegetables with one of her many blunt old knives, and I am almost too happy – for us both – to stay around in the kitchen, in case study of this miracle might scare it away.

I am upstairs, then, when the smell of soup finds me and I realize she is proving one of her own truths to me – there is something very special about the scent of cooking which you have not cooked, when cooking is a lot of what you do. Boy, do I hear that now.

She's back.

The new oven, however, remains defiant. I have just about

got my head around it now. Mum shakes hers as I talk her through its ways, before stuffing the instructions in the drawer already crammed with manuals for appliances we no longer own.

*

When I get in later, Mum has tried the oven. What she cooked was inedible, she says.

'What was it?' I ask.

'I threw it on the garden.'

That she didn't even want it in the bin is saying something. All that remains is a parched baking tray and the air of regret.

'If I'd made me that I would divorce myself,' she declares.

15 December 2017

This morning I find her crying beside the washing machine. She can't remember how to switch it on. It's cold in here as well. This rickety, glass-roofed annexe and extension of the kitchen known to us as 'the sun room' is anything but in winter. I bring her back inside and she sits down, sobbing.

'I'm useless.'

She has her head in her hands. It is the most despondent I have seen her, or perhaps that she has let me see her, since her mother died, almost forty years ago.

We have tried to steer Mum away from domestic labours, but she doesn't know who she is without them. The 'safe' old person who accepts their care and all assistance quietly and dutifully is, here at least, an external fantasy. Something we project. If you saw my mother trying to do things, you too would try to take them off her and help. But she is hanging on to something more fundamental than the iron, the shopping and the car keys. How do you let someone so fragile but determined be themselves?

This is our conundrum. My parents have deeply different and diametrically opposed responses to old age. Mum is determined, compelled even, to go out fighting, I think. To suffer the next indignity or fall or fatal whatever whilst in the act of getting something done. Of being.

The Old Man has raised the drawbridge long before the heathen comes, and now sits waiting, as though not doing anything might raise the odds of nothing happening. And if he won't do a thing then someone else will have to. Whereas with Mum the work is in reining her in.

They are the just-about-living embodiment of what physicists and philosophers call The Irresistible Force Paradox. This is assumed to be unresolvable, but I know better. I know exactly what happened when the unstoppable force met the immovable object. They got married and had us.

16 December 2017

Whatever doubts the present conjures, Mum will return to and recount unfailingly the history of her pans.

'New York, 1957,' she announces when I reach for a certain saucepan, sole survivor of its set.

'Older than you,' she reminds me.

Though I have heard all the stories before there is (at times) something reassuring about hearing them again. The pans are a reminder of my parents' transatlantic heyday, two kids from the north making a go of it on steamships, long before I was born. It wasn't always like this. They were young.

Meantime she can manage the museum of her life just as she pleases. The jewel in the proverbial crown is her Kenwood mixer. Unused of late but still sitting proudly in a place of great significance, as if it might be recalled to action any time. Another fifties relic. Another survivor. Too heavy for her to lift now but still foundation stone of her faculties, it seems, and the wellspring of many of mine. I recall flavour born from its bowl. The taste of dough dispensed ahead of baking. Sugar and some deeper sweetness fused forever in one's mind. Against this mesh of memory I watch her triumph over small things. The oven, though, still gets the evil eye.

The Naked and the Dad

I am halfway down the stairs when Mum lurches from the bathroom with several toothbrushes and a pressing question.

'Are any of these yours?'

Between the banisters I glimpse, or just allow myself to see, that she is naked. This is new – her naked, not the nakedness itself. Dad spearheaded that months ago.

From Mum, however, it is an innovation, or whatever the reverse of that may be. This is not an emergency, the toothbrush question. If it plays as one to her, however, then perhaps we have a problem. Decades of discretion undone by fears about dental hygiene. What does this say about her state of mind?

What I am also seeing but not wanting to admit here is that as Mum's outlook worsens, my parents are becoming more and more the same. It is not so much that I am in danger of losing an ally here (though that is worrying), but that the stages of decline seem to erase the individual.

'Are these yours?' she asks again. 'Or are they mine?'

The Naked and the Dad

18 December 2017

While their selves are merging and their friends are dying out, a decent haul of Christmas cards tumbles onto the mat each morning. Some of this is down to dutiful offspring who manage the seasonal post of their less capable folks. We are not there yet, at least. Mum can still write; I do the posting. We set the cards around the hearth and admire the scene.

The cards function like the old things in the kitchen. They tell my parents who they are, who cares, and where they once were together. Will our generation's screens and digital assistants offer us the same?

'Siri, who am I, and where have I been?'

One card propels Mum down memory lane, but this is no stroll. Behind the glittered robins and the Bible kings she treads a path of ancient grievance. The note comes from an old neighbour who says her husband is now too ill to drive. Mum explains this with an unfamiliar smile.

'He mocked me,' she recalls of the now immobile man. 'For learning to drive in an automatic. This was 1968.'

She looks off into the distance, half a century of deferred justice dancing in her eyes.

'Now he's not going anywhere.'

Talk about a dish served cold.

'Learning to drive and having children were the best things I ever did,' she announces.

I am proud of her, if somewhat shocked by the duration of her vengeance. I am also mindful and a little sad that these, her most beloved accomplishments, kids and car skills, have not been among mine.

'Their daughter is a dog walker!' she adds maniacally, finishing the letter.

'What's wrong with that?' I counter, dog walking being something I had tacitly considered as a career move. I mean, why not, where's the harm in it? You just—

'A DOG WALKER!'

I go upstairs and lie down. It's 11 a.m.

Sweet Emotion

I decide to make Christmas official and put some decorations up. Mum and Dad don't seem bothered, but I clamber to the attic where the symbols of good cheer are stored.

Before I hit the tinsel I am confronted with the loft's more painful legacies. Up here is where our family's failed marriages reside. Pictures of mine and my sister's weddings, thirty-five years and a thousand miles apart but united by divorce, are up here gathering dust together.

It's a progressive relegation, from the pantheon of happy pictures on permanent display in the kitchen to the rafters of regret, but the surprise still eats at my insides. The decorations seem suddenly ridiculous. I leave a smiling snowman, whose apparent happiness seems especially repugnant, behind.

Downstairs Dad's gout is worsening. He doesn't say this, instead just wincing when he puts his foot down and finding ways to move less. I examine his feet. His socks of choice are relics from hospital. Red, elasticated, with a rubberized non-slip sole. Just as he depends on and demands the red socks (which serve instead of shoes), so my mother has come to resent them.

'When I see those go on,' she laments, 'I know we're not going anywhere.'

I peel back his socks and try to remember how bad things were last time I looked. Hard to say. I have done the online diligence, googled the gout. The tophi themselves are not a problem. My brain might not want to look upon them, but his body doesn't seem to mind. Dad's fresh pain on walking is not necessarily a part of this.

God knows there is enough other stuff going on. I have had consultants describe his array of illnesses as 'a puzzle', 'a balancing act' and, simply, 'complex'. Some other painful part of him or problem might have descended to his feet just to announce itself.

Either way, they hurt. He can't fit a slipper, let alone a shoe, and though he loves the hospital socks as much as his wife hates them, they will not do. There is but one place we can go for help. Back to our sacred river and provider: Amazon.

He stabs the screen. I man the door. Pairs come and we try to squeeze them on. We fail, and then my sister returns them. This rinses and repeats. I fashion some spiritual amnesty that stops me getting pissed off about how often I must get up and answer the door. Pain in his toes keeping me on mine.

Let loose upon the tablet he runs wild, and even more weird crap than usual makes its way down the drive. Mad Santa. Three massive, duty-free-size Toblerones come in three separate deliveries. The place is so hot that they wilt like joke-shop wands as soon as they arrive.

'I thought I was just buying one normal one,' he says defensively.

Sweet Emotion

The house is as much a swollen, diabetic nightmare as his lower limbs. Each cupboard bursts with biscuits and chocolate like some schoolboy stash. Why, then, I am compelled to ask him, would we need a Toblerone of any size, at all?

'I thought it would be a change,' he confesses.

Oddly, suddenly, and all too briefly, I unambiguously love him for that.

★

Still the slipper suitors come, each bringing a pair wider than the last until the pantomime 'Gouterella' concludes with the arrival of a Velcro-flapped pair broad enough to set sail in. He is briefly reborn in them. There is a nasty, red-yellow tinge to the tophi now.

'Let's keep an eye on it,' I say, and we agree on this fudge, master and pupil of avoidance.

Back into the kitchen. A large Scotch. More biscuits. I make the gout speech, though I'm not convinced it, or anything else, even matters any more.

20 December 2017

Days ago my sister-in-law bought Dad a fancy scallop dish from Marks & Spencer. I feel enough like a prison guard (and just as trapped as my inmates) that I don't clamp down on outside food. But the Old Man has now become obsessed with it.

'Do you want a cup of tea?'

'Can I have the scallops?'

'What shall we do today?'

'Can you get those scallops?'

I told him they don't have it at the shops we go to (true). He ordered several online. Today they arrive in separate deliveries. So many I can scarcely fit them in the freezer. Mum gets angry.

'One was enough!'

I don't like scallops. Don't really know how to cook them. Don't like the look of them. Mum rustles up the frozen ones carefully if resentfully. Stuffed to the gills with spineless snacks I leave them to it, run up to London for therapy and to visit an old friend with a new baby born seven weeks premature.

His daughter is not much bigger than my hand. Her eyes are clamped shut and her body is pulsing, curled up like she is still in the womb, or wishes she were. I know the feeling. Her Dad and I worked in nightclubs together, but here we are now. One punter in too soon at his door. Two that won't leave at mine. I wonder if this all adds up somewhere. One in, one out.

Corruption and Eruption

Before I head home, I squeeze in a Christmas party. People I've worked with over the years ask me difficult questions about where I've been. I answer, and spin the anecdotes I've honed at Dave's and elsewhere into set pieces. A good friend takes me aside and says –

'This stuff is important. You should be writing it down.'

'I am. A bit,' I tell him. 'I don't know what else to do.'

'Write more. Get it organized. Show someone.'

22 December 2017

As well as writing, I take refuge in books. Without even trying I find myself learning about the Aché, Paraguayan hunter-gatherers who kill one another when they get weak or old. In the account I have they seem a little trigger-happy. Children that don't appear to make the grade are dispatched too. Still, as is often the case when acquainted with aboriginal wisdom, I look about me and wonder if what we have inflicted on ourselves and all the world is really progress.

My fellow feeling with the Aché is compounded by the temperature here, akin to the Paraguayan rainforest, carpet notwithstanding. I must get away again before I lapse into a loincloth and kill.

Another food delivery is due. They can argue over the mad bounty without me. Even if all they get is ham and toilet paper, they'll survive. It's like opening several tins of cat food, I tell myself. If they don't like it they will go and miaow next door, perhaps. Or eat one another. I am past caring.

I'm almost out of the door for another night in London when I am struck by an arrow from the jungle. Dad calls.

'Something's happened.'

The arrow is poison-tipped. The type of toxin where madness precedes death.

'It's my foot.'

Is it ever. The gamey, yellow-puce king-tophi on the right has burst. Lumps of what look like chalk, but which are presumably crystals of uric acid, are flowing out on a stream of pus from a hole in the toe. We should go to the doctor. But Dad refuses to move.

I subdue my inner tribesman and get on the phone. First to the doctors, then to the person I was hoping to get drunk with. An outcall GP can take several hours to arrive. I go back to my books. Dad, though shocked at what is emerging from his body, doesn't appear to be in too much pain.

The doctor is a handsome man in a Barbour jacket. I am so pleased to have someone who isn't old or a blood relative to talk to that it takes a while before the grim truth dawns that he is younger than me. I am at that point in my depression, life, or whatever this is, when every other living thing and even some inanimate objects appear to have made better choices than me.

Doc Barbour is polite, disarming. He notes Dad's maritime memorabilia and they get chatting about the sea. It is all convivial until he presses Dad's toe and then the Old Man flinches. This flinch is the fastest I have ever seen him move and so it follows that the pain from this is through the roof. I have an outbreak of sympathy.

'It is infected,' the physician deduces. I nod, patiently, like I am the authority in the room.

He squeezes an unholy trail of matter from the wound, sterilizes and dresses it. I assist. We chat. I drop some technical terms I've learned along the way: 'tophi', 'debridement'.

'Have you had medical training?' he asks. Twisting the knife of what might have been.

'No,' I say. 'Just don't have much else to do at the moment.'

'Well, you seem to understand what's going on here.'

'Yeah . . .'

I am reminded of a character in *Apocalypse Now* who, when asked if he knows who is in command of an anarchic jungle outpost, just growls in the affirmative and disappears into the darkness. I snap out of cinematic fantasy as I am handed a prescription: oral antibiotics.

'Might shift it,' says the doctor. 'Let us know if he gets diarrhoea.'

He doesn't sound optimistic. He is leaving, however, and that looks exciting. I think about asking him for a lift to the chemist, but worry that I might claim sanctuary and refuse to leave the car. Perhaps I'll stow away in the boot while he's talking to Dad. Instead, I cycle to the pharmacy. On the way, the bike collapses.

Stop the Calvary

23 December 2017

Back at the house I dig out an old plastic sleeve that we used last time someone couldn't get their foot wet and needed to shower.

'I just won't bother,' says Dad when I present the appendage.

The climate of defeat is lifted briefly by the arrival of my brother and his youngest daughter. Mum is sufficiently emboldened by this that she agrees to visit her oldest nearby friend, Florence, Bill's widow. Since this constitutes progress and because I think I am going insane here, I go along for the ride. It is less than half a mile away.

It is great to see Mum and her former neighbour chatting. Kids and professionals might help, but there's nothing like an old friend. I take a picture of them talking and send it to her son, my friend from early childhood. These images are helpful among the network of absent children; we trade them when they come. It's good just to see something that merits a photograph.

'It's helpful in old age,' her friend says, 'to have a wide range of interests.'

'Migraines and incest?' says Mum, without a hint of contrivance. She fiddles with her hearing aid as we laugh but is happy to see us doing so.

'What did I say?' she asks knowingly.

'MIGRAINES AND INCEST!' we answer, more than once, until the joke is clear.

I don't remember when this many of us had this much fun. It is like old times.

24 December 2017

The plan is that tomorrow my brother will drive us out to his place for lunch. This is anticipated here with the stoic formality of those going on a possibly fatal mission. Like a squadron conscious of both risk and duty, we await the dawn.

The tension is too much for me and I take refuge in the reliable respite of a long walk with John and his dog. I feel like a fraud and a fuck-up, convinced I shouldn't be out among the living, that every other dog and walker on the path has a better life and a clearer heart than mine. That said, I question whether we kid ourselves on that level. For sure, we have different opportunities, but choices? I wonder if we choose at all.

I'm uncertain what it says about my character, but my fatalistic funk is entirely dispelled when the dog, an aged but tenacious Jack Russell, attempts to attack an eagle owl which is being paraded in front of children singing carols at a garden centre.

We further lighten the mood by watching the full 149-minute

German-language version of *Das Boot*. It might be my parents who lived through the war, but I feel I can relate to the stench, claustrophobia and pending threat of life on a U-Boat. I walk home drunk, wondering if I am too old to join the armed forces.

Merry Gentlemen

25 December 2017

I wake up wondering why it should be that I would rather be on a maritime mission than stepping through the festivities with my family. I used to love Christmas. Today feels like forced labour at the cracker factory. It's tempting to recall that oceanic excursions were exactly what kept my dad from being around at Christmas when I was young, but despite the appealing symmetry, such a judgement is unfair. I have made my own mess. And it *has* given me a secret mission. Get through today without bursting into tears or punching anyone in the face.

It is the time of miracles, and so it comes to pass that my parents both make it to my brother's for lunch and back again and I don't do anything mental. We don't stay long but the ceremony is complete, the generations gathered for an hour or two. Like sovereigns of some forgotten state shuffling out onto the balcony and waving to a crowd, it seems astonishing they still wield power. The part of me that wants a revolution surrenders briefly to the part of me content to smile and wave back.

My nephew has given my mum an electric blanket. In an

object lesson in each other's opposite world views, Mum is delighted but the Old Man rails against it.

'You can go up in flames,' he reckons.

I have a thousand retorts for that, but let it slide. I fit the blanket. By the time I've finished everyone is asleep anyway. I have a substantial whisky and join them on the other side.

26 December 2017

I am within sight of the unoccupied bathroom when Dad calls me to his bedroom. I note the things upon his chest of drawers. Hymns for his funeral. A note saying he no longer wishes to donate his organs to science and a famous speech from Shakespeare about England: 'This fortress built by Nature for herself / Against infection and the hand of war . . .'

Nature has plans of her own, however. Infection, too. The dressing is off his toe and what lies beneath is grisly.

I clean it up as best I can and reattach the dressing. The district nurse is due tomorrow, I think. No sense rattling the system on Boxing Day. Dad's guts have, as ever, their own agenda and the doctor's diarrhoea prophecy is soon upon us. No more antibiotics. And no more arguments about having a shower.

I fit the plastic leg sleeve and steer him into the cubicle where he clings grimly to the grab rail as the water descends. I look at myself in the mirror. Comfortably the youngest in the room but still heading in the wrong direction. When I was growing up this room was lit by a fluorescent tube which spared me nothing of my erupting teenage complexion. If you looked OK under that light you probably looked amazing elsewhere. That, at least, was the theory.

'How is it under there?' I ask him.

'Wonderful,' he says.

Despite everything, this is the highlight of the season. The small victories are getting even smaller, but their power remains.

Afterwards, Dad does not wish to go downstairs, and returns to bed understandably drained. Mum isn't up to much either. I take them toast and watch TV alone in the living room with the window open, which feels like freedom somehow. Mum rises eventually. Dad just goes to the bathroom, sleeps and eats. I have plans for the evening. The deferred night out is back on.

*

Dave and I head to a bar run by another friend of ours which is having a soul night. This has become a reliable Boxing Day fixture for those of us you might call Thatcher's children.

When the bar shuts, we form a gang with other middle-aged strays and head over to what was once a cinema but is now a vast, obnoxious nightclub.

'Don't you know who I was?' I blurt to the bouncers.

They eventually let us in.

My drink, whatever it is, shudders to the beat. Tinnitus will be in overdrive tomorrow. The plastic glass, the iceless beverage, the pulsing, limbic sound erase all pasts, recent and recalled.

Then I feel my phone shudder. I shudder too, back into reality. It is 2 a.m. My parents' number. There is nothing good on the end of this call, and no way in here to hear what's being said. Whatever it is, the only thing to do will be to go straight home or directly to the hospital.

If it's the hospital then someone is already in safe hands. Home it is. Sobriety rinses through me on the back of adrenaline. I say goodbye to everyone, point to the phone and mouth, 'Mum and Dad'.

I get into a taxi without calling back and tell him to drive me home. I ready myself for whatever has happened there.

I can cope.

We can cope.

A human being can get through anything.

I repeat this until I almost believe it. I am surprised, when we head down the hill and I can see the house, that there is not a single light on.

I expected, perhaps even wanted, an ambulance. Maybe one has been and gone. Maybe they are both inside it. Dad's special reading lamp, the kind of broadsheet offer that has the elderly in its cross hairs, emits a light so bright you have to squint as you look at the house. It's like a star gate, a portal, a tear in the fabric of time. At least he can read the paper, even if you need a welding mask to take him a cup of tea. Had that been on I could probably have seen it from town. The Dad signal, stretched bright across the firmament. Instead, the dark.

I let myself in and call hello. Mum wouldn't hear me whatever had happened. I see Dad's light go on upstairs and run into his bedroom.

'What's going on?'

'I just . . .' he seems confused. He is holding the phone from which he must have called me, 'wondered where you were.'

What follows requires some qualification. I hope I make no judgement here, but my father has never in my adult life, as I recollect, phoned me just to see where I am, or how I am. Which is not to say those things have never crossed his mind. Far from it.

'I thought you might have been mugged,' he adds.

I have, I think to myself. By you.

I believe him in the literal sense. What I question, I confess, is the degree to which the outcome of any mugging might have been assessed in terms of his immediate well-being, as opposed to mine. Most of all, though, I am back here, at the very heart and hearth of the place I sought to flee. Abducted and recalled for what seems to me, right now, to be no good reason. I am also brimming with suppressed panic and cheap booze. As I stand there in his room all this coalesces into anger, which makes itself known.

27 December 2017

I don't know what I said or how loudly, but I awake sore-headed with a sense that Dad looked scared. I know how bad things can get when I get mean. My life has many of these mornings. Hot with guilt, I go downstairs, where Mum is rattling about. Her vibe is off. You never know the subtle emanations of a household until they go askew.

I try to explain what I was feeling, but she shakes her head, which is worse than her not hearing. She is sick of it today, I think: me, him, us. Everything.

'This isn't what I signed up for,' she will say in her most despondent moments.

I can never hear that without resolving to amend the problem. Seldom do I believe (or can I even bear to think) that the problem might be me.

I go upstairs to see Dad. Pains in my guts, head, heart from multiple sources. Maybe we can make something of this, have a proper talk. He is in bed, doing the looking-away thing.

'I'm sorry,' I say.

I move in and try to embrace him. He allows that. It becomes a sort of hug. He is rigid in my arms. Sheets and more between us. Something in him can't or won't respond to me. Then he speaks.

'I can't breathe,' he says.

No, you can't, can you. I let him go. He points at a box of the incontinence pants he favours.

'Those say absorbent,' he explains. 'I want the ones that say protective.'

You and me both, mate. Back to it, then.

Requiem for a Middleweight

Now Dad can't walk on the infected foot, so we hobble together to the bathroom and back to his bed, a short enough journey. I make and take him food. Mum is coming downstairs more often now, but it is a diminished version of the woman we knew. If she speaks it's to ask a question about what she has just done. She can't read, concentrate or relax and so is restless and unhappy, a tough combination at any time of life. One of them is always too hot, the other too cold. They call out for me so often, Dad especially, that I start to twitch at the sound of my own name. The house is stifling. The plumbing groans as if it too were in pain.

I do the things I do when I can get out. Dog walks. Visit Dave and his young, exuberant son, which feels curative yet oddly poignant. There are days when young lives rattle the ghosts of what I have not done with mine.

29 December 2017

My friend Lennie, whose mother died of cancer earlier this year, is slowly clearing out their place. He comes and gets me in her car and cooks an astounding meal. He lived in Italy for a time and makes great food. Pasta apart, there is a natural sadness to what he's doing. Shutting up shop on his childhood, a house we've both known.

I think about people who've been through these bereavements. I've seen them front it out, necessarily so under logistical burdens, the fixers of this world, and then pay later. I talk with one who tells me she recorded every sound of every door and cupboard and space before she left her childhood home. That feels like something I might do. I'm not one for clean breaks. I need a souvenir.

Inspired by Lennie, I try and make Mum some pasta, but make the mistake of asking her which kind she'd like while she is having a deaf moment.

'What is it?' she asks.

Linguine, I answer.

'What?'

Linguine.

'What?'

LINGUINE!

'*What?*'

LINGUINE!

'What?'

I start slapping myself in the face with a packet of salmon at this point, like some kind of performance art.

LINGUINE! (SMACK) LINGUINE! (SMACK) LINGUINE!

'Oh, do calm down,' says Mum.

30 December 2017

Dad's whole foot turns red. I call the surgery. They send a doctor and I lead her upstairs to the Old Man. She takes the dressing off his toe and pulls a face. I feel a surge of pride. It's good to know I'm not worn out by anything banal.

'What would you say . . .' she asks him, 'about a trip to hospital?'

What floods into me at that point dwarfs the previous pride. If he was in hospital we could relax a little. Focus more on Mum. Or just do nothing. What floods into me in that fraction of a second, before he speaks, is hope.

'No,' he says. 'Not hospital,' looking genuinely afraid.

My hope wanes. I know what this will mean.

We try to persuade him. He won't have any of it. She concedes. Instead, a district nurse will come every three days and check the wound. I explain that the dressings don't stay on. Too much stuff is coming out. I have to keep cleaning it and redressing it.

'Are you happy to keep doing that?'

I make a gesture which is as close to 'no' as a positive can get.

She switches him to a stronger antibiotic. Bad news for his guts and my oversight of their output.

'I can still have a Scotch,' he states, rhetorically.

She frowns.

'How much does he drink?'

Again, I make a conflicted gesture.

'You're on a lot of pills,' she says. 'It won't help.'

Then something astonishing happens. She is sitting on the

bed; he is propped up in it. He starts bobbing and weaving like a boxer, playfully swinging at her like an entreating child.

'Lemme have a drink!' he says. His voice is weirdly pitiful, contrived but heartfelt, somehow.

'Lemme have a drink, go on . . .'

I realize then, and it will stay and build in me throughout the coming days and settle like some toxic mud, that I have never seen him like this before. Playful, physical. I don't remember that growing up, much as I might have wished to.

That he can't consider what his intransigence inflicts on the rest of us . . . I feel stunned. Insulted. Sick, empty, lonely and sad. I don't even remember what the doctor says. Don't care. All my life I wanted some example from a man who wasn't there. Now here we are, and this is it. My therapist says accommodations made in infancy are buried deep, before language and conscious memory, even. Whatever I have buried, the ruins are rising today.

I believe the technical phrase for where we are is 'proximal separation'. We have never been physically closer, but I have never felt further away. I file my feelings and press on.

'How are you for the old LSD?' asks Mum, as we eat dinner.

She means money, in the pounds, shillings and pence format, but I have to laugh. Hallucinogens might help me more than cash this evening. But there will be no more doctors here today.

You think you have conquered certain fears, but life has a way of finding us out. I felt I could clean up anything, but what emerges and keeps emerging from Dad's abscess tonight takes me to the limits of repulsion.

I squeeze out his poison and swallow my own.

Elder Skelter

31 December 2017

In a nightmare I hear wailing. But the sound persists and I awaken, aware that this is real. It's Dad's voice, coming from the bathroom. He isn't calling anyone's name or crying for help. It's just a painful sound.

I can force the door just enough to see his legs behind it. He must have fallen and now lies against the door, jamming it shut. Even the few inches I can crack it are quickly reclaimed as he squirms towards me, getting nowhere. This was one of his stated fears. I had considered reversing the hinges so it opened outwards, but had no idea how to go about that, and so it got sidelined, and now here we are.

'Can you move?'

He says my name as a question. I push the door, almost edging in, but he wails and I retreat. I know the right thing to do is call 999. If the paramedics come there is a good chance he will go to hospital, get fixed up and we can take a breather. Instead, acting against everyone's interests including, and perhaps especially, my own, I shove the door despite his lowing protest, and slip through the gap into the bathroom.

Inside it's like a crime scene. He is sprawled on the pale-blue tiles in a kind of foetal curl around the base of the toilet. His catheter and the long tube that leads to his night bag – the likely culprit for this fall – are tangled about his legs, one of which is bleeding.

'Where am I?' he asks.

I try to lift him but can't.

'You have to help me,' I say. 'Give me something.'

Little by little, he starts to push. It's enough of a boost that I manage to heave him up onto the toilet.

'What happened?'

'I think you fell. Maybe we should call someone?'

'No. No way.'

I wash and dress his leg wound. He doesn't seem to be in any pain, nor does he appear to be entirely conscious. After a few minutes I help him back to the bedroom.

By morning he has no memory of what happened. The dressing is coming off his foot, however, and he'd like a cup of tea. Life goes on, even in its most depleted measure.

Soon enough we are back in the bathroom and draining the abscess. I have overcome my revulsion by becoming obsessive about the quality of the dressing, cutting ever more careful bandages each time. Indignity and inconvenience apart, we aren't having that bad a time, I tell myself. It is a good thirty-minute ritual, this. At some point he will apologize for everything.

'I'm sorry,' he says.

'I don't mind,' I answer. I believe we mean it, too.

I do however spill so much TCP on his bedroom carpet that the smell makes me weep, and no amount of cleaning will shift it. Dad seems immune to this somehow, or at least he will not allow me to open a window to shift the cloud of antiseptic vapour. The stench lingers.

★

Mum is a picnic, comparatively speaking. Still shadow-Mum, but independent at least. She runs her frail dominion. There is no talk of going anywhere. Except from me.

I take a walk as the sun sets mid afternoon. By the time I am heading back there are already fireworks. I think of all the New Year's parties I have been to, and watch lights exploding in the sky from parties I will never know.

I have to get out of here.

I call Dave. His partner is a midwife, working a night shift. He will be in, his youngest asleep. I head over there, and we drink. Before midnight he is asleep on the sofa. I look at him and the pictures of his family.

I walk home and tell myself that life is what we make it at any given moment, not an accumulation of things and check-points that add up to some distant win, or hollow failure. Whatever it is, this is it.

1 January 2018

Mornings are becoming more elaborate. The clinical rituals – drain and dress the abscess (now bigger than the toe), drain the catheter bag, get Dad back to bed then fetch up breakfast, meanwhile check Mum – are becoming more routine. If they are both fed and stable by midday and I have had a shower, then that's a good day.

Elder Skelter

Before sunset I take Mum for a stilted but much-needed totter around the block. The angle of the hill and the accumulation of moss on the frost-broken pavements make this treacherous, even for me. Mum is stir-crazy, if one can say such a thing about someone who is also, by their standards, depressed. It takes a while. It would be quicker and easier to carry her, but that's not the point.

We're a hundred metres from the front door but I feel like I'm showing her around. I like it. This is proper old-people stuff. Fresh air, memories, interdependence. This I can do.

We turn back into our road. The house glows ahead, still homely but with an air of foreboding. In there anything can happen, and something is coming, I can feel it. Something must break or burst or change. Or I will.

Out here in the dusk, under the leafless trees where my imagination would once have sown all kinds of fears, now this feels like safety. It has become so difficult indoors that I would sooner be an outsider, sometimes.

Grace Under Pressure

2 January 2018

The district nurse is scheduled, so I take extra care to make Dad's dressing neat. If this is what I do now I want praise from an expert. Acknowledgement that if this is my life, then at least I am good at it. Or not too bad, or something. If I stray outside the moment, the unknown future, the rueful past, are worse than what is taking place right now. In this mess, for all its undesirability, I know who I am. I know that I am needed. It is an identity, even if it is not a costume I would have chosen. I came late to the superhero meeting. All the best ones had gone.

I tell myself I am 'good', but in truth I am failing. Coming apart. I need drugs to sleep and drink to be awake, some days. The place is full of both. My internal breakdown is ever outstripped by the continuous slide of my father's faculties. He's getting weaker, or less interested, or both. His foot looks as if it's been in a fire. The redness is rising past his ankle, up his leg. We sit on the edge of his bed and survey the damage. Will he go to hospital now?

'No,' he says. Defiant.

I slope downstairs and make him breakfast. The papers and

TV run stories of the annual winter beds crisis. Operations are cancelled, and patients are left in corridors. This seems to worsen daily. Maybe he wouldn't even qualify under these conditions. The doctor's offer to admit him seems a lifetime ago. He's scared. Mum is miserable. I am angry. While sepsis chews the toes, fear eats the soul.

I go up and down the stairs so many times this morning that I feel insane. Dad and I both love the movie *Cool Hand Luke*, which is, in a certain analysis, a hymn to being stubborn and charismatically, self-destructively defiant. At one point the titular hero is tasked by sadistic prison guards with digging a hole and then filling it back up again. This continues until he is physically, if not quite spiritually, broken. Though it is my father who is digging his fetid heels in to avoid what he perceives as prison, it is I, his valet, who is beginning to crumble at the endless back and forth. I have come apart before, so I know what it feels like. Something in me is ringing like an alarm.

Downtime becomes so scarce that sometimes I just stand still. I am doing this in the hall, a liminal space between the possible future of the dining room (where I gaze at the Internet) and the presenting past of my bedroom (where I sift through drawers of adolescent tat) and the rest of the house's loaded bases, when there is a knock at the front door.

I startle, as though this was unexpected gunfire. Another sign I'm losing it. I can hear Mum making the 'ugh' sound that means she is trying to stand up or move something heavy. Even lifting her handbag prompts this now. The 'ugh' is somewhere between James Brown in an exuberant mood and a death metal artist in a bad one. A remarkable thing for a woman her size, but still a call to arms if one is within earshot.

'I'll get it,' I shout, and open the door.

The district nurse. Not one of the team I recognize, but a welcome sight. I have seen enough health care professionals over the threshold now that I know better than to idolize them. They are as prone to moods and madness as the rest of us; more so, maybe, given their terrain. Nevertheless, this young woman looks me in the eye kindly and I am infused with calm. Faith, even. Maybe I don't have to figure all this out for myself.

'Where is your father?' she asks.

I dig the drama of her question. We could be starring in any number of movies now. I show her upstairs, rattling off the symptoms and laying out the scene.

I talk. He talks. The nurse nods and listens. I want her to notice how carefully I have bandaged his foot, but she is in a rhythm of her own as she unwraps it.

She swabs the leaking wound and strokes the spreading redness which is rising toward his thigh. The foot is puce. I show her the antibiotics and the rest of the regimen. Relay the last conversation with the doctor. Then she says the most amazing thing.

'You need to go to hospital.'

Dad counterpunches. Flat out refuses, but this woman has a way about her. He makes his protests, 'The doctor said . . .' She kindly but firmly disarms him. I am ready to back her up, primed with the kind of aimless positive chatter we put out when accompanying another to the scaffold, but I can see he is out of moves and I can also see his fear.

It makes no earthly sense for him to be here. It is squeezing the life out of all of us to look after him. But in his mind hospital is worse. He is resolutely of the 'once you go in, you'll never come out' school of thought. I point out he has been in and made it home four times this year. He has had more comebacks than Elvis, even if he doesn't want to die like him. Now Vegas is calling once again. But the King doesn't like the odds.

'No,' he says.

'Dad . . .' I say.

Mum calls from downstairs. The nurse motions me to leave. I forget what Mum needs, probably just an update or a reminder of something said before. I am on my way back upstairs again, when I am struck hard by the weight of everything. A mouse in a clock, hit by the pendulum.

The everyday vibration of not knowing which way to turn accelerates into something beyond outer sound or inner feeling. A molecular shift which prevents me moving any closer to my father's room, as if the emotional reality were now some physical barrier. I sink to my knees as best one can on a stair-case. The heating clanks on methodically but in all other aspects of perception, time stills.

Across the stair carpet, dappled light spills from the window of my old bedroom. Out of its pattern something sublime dismantles my despair, and grace, if you will, enters in.

I know then, and not in the normal way of learning but in some more fundamental and freeing sense, that whatever happens next, what I do or do not do, does not ultimately matter. And there is enough energy in this realization that I can stand up, go back, past blame and recrimination and on into the bedroom. This is beyond me, and that's OK. The nurse looks up at me and says –

'He will go.'

*

We always have a bag ready. Pyjamas, money, phone and charger. Book, toothbrush, comb and radio. I fetch it. I move as if I am dreaming, in shock from the reprieve. I take nothing for granted. He is going to be examined, not admitted. No guarantee we even get a night off.

'There are no beds,' he says, quoting the newspaper.

'That tells you how serious this is. How important you are. No one,' I add, 'is doing this for fun.'

Getting him into the hospital is a considerable manoeuvre and my respect for the nurse turns to unmitigated wonder as she goes about this. She runs multiple and simultaneous conversations between the GP, the hospital microbiology unit, the ambulance service and the hospital admissions team.

She builds an HQ at our kitchen table, filling out paperwork and working from our landline while ignoring her own mobile, which rings constantly if she is not making an outgoing call. It's her supervisor, she explains, urging her to move on to the next job. Her demeanour is calm and constant. When there is a break in the proceedings, she looks across at me and asks me how I am.

With this simple question the entire construct of my coping collapses and I find myself fighting tears. If I wasn't leaning on the counter I might collapse. She nods, as though my inner fiction was as obvious and unsustainable as the foul state of my father's toe. It has been a while since anyone asked me how I was doing, let alone the agent of my salvation. While she is here, this unexpected saint, dispensing patient truth and justice, she gives me a share.

'Look after yourself,' she says, 'you can't do all this. Get some help here or you aren't helping anyone.'

I still want to fall over, but now in thanks, in supplication.

When everything is in place, the ambulance booked, she explains that Dad will not have to go in through A & E, which is a relief to him. She says the GP will call and confirm his admission. I am at a loss as to how to express my relief. I am trying to thank her, but she is already out of the door and talking to her supervisor, the rancour in their voice rattling through the phone. She has been here over an hour.

When the doctor rings – perhaps Dad's sparring partner from the other day – she sounds stressed. Dad will be admitted to Ambulatory Care for assessment, she says. I can tell she wants to get off the phone, but I don't like the sound of this.

'Ambulatory means walking,' I point out. 'He can't walk.'

'It doesn't mean that in this context,' she says.

But she has had the misfortune to call a pedant who has glimpsed freedom.

'Ambulatory means walking,' I repeat. 'He can't walk. He needs a bed.'

Please God keep him overnight, I almost say.

'He'll be assessed,' is all she can tell me.

We wait for the ambulance. I tell Mum what's going on and her relief is as palpable as Dad's discomfort as I tell him everything will be OK.

Dad will buck like a mule from what he fears but he is quick to make accommodation with the inevitable. When the paramedics arrive he is stoic and amiable. They fold him into a collapsible stretcher and carry him downstairs. I rush to the tiny bathroom. He can have the mirror. A gesture of thanks to him, to whatever went down back on the stairs. I stick the looking glass in the go-bag, kiss Mum goodbye and close the door.

This time we miss the high-tech wonder of the ICU and its moat of mayhem – A & E. Instead we roll calmly into the bold new terrain of Ambulatory Care or ACU. Six beds in which you wait to be assessed and where all expedient measures can be applied.

For all the headlines proclaiming otherwise, the hospital is calm. Dad is swabbed, prodded and X-rayed. His foot looks awful. People who have seen their share of shit, I'm sure, give it a double take. Again I feel pride. What a piece of work is a man. Two hours ago, I was on the edge of a nervous breakdown or a spiritual breakthrough. Now I'm considering selling tickets by my ailing father's side.

We wait on results, yet even the delay is soothing. I tell Dad to call me if anything happens and go for a wander. I greet familiar corridors like old friends. Good morning, Acute Medical Unit. Happy New Year, Cardiology.

*

Queueing for coffee, I find the context I am after. The hospital special. Here in the cafe are the megastars of misfortune. The chemo kids and the dementia-stricken elderly against whom all troubles shrivel in comparison. Unless of course those troubles are your own. For the rest of us, blessings abound.

There is a sandwich they have here that I quite like; today it tastes like heaven. No, I don't have a loyalty card, but I might be happier than I have ever been in any restaurant. Even though people here are crying, at least I didn't cause it. I get Dad a coffee and glide back through the crowd to ACU.

The doctor returns. Whatever lives in Dad's foot can only be faced down by intravenous antibiotics. That means admission. I don't punch the air or anything undignified, but I am deeply relieved.

'I accept it,' says Dad.

I am grateful for that. For all that I appear to have been touched by some supernatural strength, any further confrontation would have seen me liquefy; they could have poured my spirits down the sink here with everything else our bodies can't contain.

For all his fears, the Old Man respects authority when he perceives it, and this doctor's vibe is spot on. Bedside manner is a form of high-stakes comic timing. When it works it's wondrous. When it misses the mark I have seen Dad form abiding grudges. Equally, certain doctors are quickly deified. Today's practitioner is firmly in the beloved category. With something like serenity on my father's brow I depart. I have no memory of the journey home.

In his six-hour absence there have been multiple Amazon deliveries. I balance them into a pile, a cairn of crap upon his chair. Over the next days the deliveries will dwindle, then one day, nothing. I turn down the heating, prise open the window in the living room and breathe in the cold. For the respite of every hospital admission, there is (one hopes, mostly) a discharge. But then we must adapt to some fresh and perhaps accelerated regimen and learn our world all over again. When it's hard just to keep things stable, even progress can feel like a kick in the teeth. Mum makes it downstairs and asks me what will happen next. It has been a long time since I could answer that question.

All we can say is, something will.

Under the Knife

With Dad in hospital I sleep more easily, but the days remain fraught with things to do. Visiting him is chief among them. If I borrow my sister's clown bike, I can make the trip in fifteen minutes. It's a measure of Dad's pragmatism that he cites proximity to the hospital as one of the things he likes about the house, which only raises the suspicion that he had this morbid masterplan mapped out forty years ago like some fiendish general. Or perhaps that's what being sensible is like. I wouldn't know. What I do know is that this at least is different from the days before and that alone feels bracing.

I aim to see him twice a day. If I get there in time for the doctor's rounds then I get a summary of the situation first-hand. If Dad must relay it to me then there will be mistakes and confusion. Information is not necessarily power in these situations, but it offers something like sanity. An explanation, at least. Without an advocate he would be lost in here. A ghost cowed by the machine.

He is on a vascular ward since the non-healing of his foot is as much down to the woeful state of the blood vessels serving it as to the opportunistic infections that have taken up residence there. Dad is scheduled for an angioplasty, in which a balloon is fed into a blood vessel and inflated to expand it and then a stent is inserted to maintain it. But in the beds crisis, cancellations are rife.

Meantime Dad is relatively chipper since at least he is not on the geriatric wards he has come to fear. His ward mates, many due for or recovering from amputations, are younger than him. Some are younger than me. There is a high percentage of former sailors up here, not surprising given the nature of our city.

One, freshly one-legged, unvisited and in his thirties, decides that I am the best person to buy him sweets and cigarettes, diet and addiction doing to him what decades of military service could not. There is a lot of that in here, it appears to me. Conditions one might consider self-inflicted, but the selves doing the infliction are shaped by different shades of poverty; experiential, financial, loneliness or just bad luck.

7 January 2018

Mum too has seized on the mind/body connection and self-diagnosed.

'I have learnt a new word,' she announces. 'And the word is "stress".'

In Dad's absence she has been quietly rebuilding herself, like some deep AI or unknown species impervious to weapons. Now she is back, and reading articles about stress in the news-paper.

'Stress is what I've got.'

When she finds something she likes in the news she will run with it, syndicating the story repeatedly in the regional paper of her mind.

'People have started realizing they need proper breakfasts!' she shouts at me one morning, wielding the front page.

Perhaps a veiled attack on my own vegetarianism but more likely a rebuttal of modern trends. I have even been warned off eating poppy seed bagels by her since these, apparently, mean that you test positive for heroin. The list goes on.

But with stress she is on to something. I feel it just being here. I can't imagine what it does to her, forty years and three worrisome kids down the line. I prefer not to. The sense that my mother's well-being is collateral damage in the fight for my father's survival, or just his mission to stay at home, is more than I can handle.

I convene with Mum and my siblings. I quote the district nurse. We need proper help at home. It emerges that this has been the fleeting but felt consensus for some time. Through being here I am enabling a level of denial around certain realities which is wrapped in denials of my own. There is a certain co-dependency to caring. It doesn't take long before you don't know who you are, and I was in trouble with all that anyway.

Though we are glad of the respite, the source of Dad's admission (gout, enabled by a side order of diabetes) stirs old resentments in the camp. I get (and indeed have felt) the passing joy of blame. But what good does it do us in the here and now?

Everyone lets off steam to everyone else about everyone

else. This is spoken of positively as 'venting', but it appears to me we are just passing the parcel of our own exasperation in some endless, painful game. We have, like many families, come to function this way. One day Mum gets up a huge head of angst about Dad and I am forced to pull away.

'Do not,' I announce theatrically, 'make me a vessel for your complaints.'

I share this exchange with my sister. She says she wishes she'd said that thirty years ago. You learn a lot in this foxhole, it turns out. All the same, there has to be a better way.

I change his sheets and tidy his room, which is still alive with the scent of TCP. Once accustomed to the smell I stay and survey the things that matter to him. Odd souvenirs, that handwritten letter explaining that on no account does he want his body to be left to science, news which will break some hearts at the gout museum, I'm sure.

I get the measure of the house without him, shift the Amazon obelisk and sit in his chair. It is comfortable. I can see why he is loath to leave it.

Notices about Norovirus and unnecessary visits forestall any discussion of Mum going to see him. Instead they share a nightly phone call, or the version of that when one participant is quite deaf and the other has little to say.

It is sweet, in its way. After all this time they still care enough to say good night to one another. On the distant planet of old age, far from the sun of youth, politeness is important, it seems to me.

Waiting for The Man

9 January 2018

Though remote, Dad remains adept at finding things for us to do. My mobile phone breaks and I call the hospital so they can tell him not to call me on it. He doesn't answer his own mobile or read texts; it is strictly a summons-issuing machine. He rings me on the landline at 9 p.m. It's late. I'm primed for big news. Let's hear it . . .

'I need a biro.'

'Now?'

There's a pause while he thinks this through.

'Tomorrow.'

'I'll buy one at the hospital.'

'No. Bring one from the house.'

10 January 2018

'I'm having a vasectomy,' he tells me the next morning, pen in hand. A pen he already had.

Vascular surgery, he means. We laugh, but when the hour approaches he falls solemn as the risk of general anaesthetic is explained. I listen, thinking this would not be a bad way to go. Perhaps he thinks this too. We say nothing, so we'll never know. They wheel him away to theatre and I go for a walk.

When the novelty of being in hospital subsides I spend a lot of time here waiting for him to wake up, be washed, or endure some new procedure; consequently I wander the halls like a ghost until I need a place here to hide. To this end I find myself in the hospital chapel, the only unbranded, non-medical place in the whole mammoth institution. If you are not on a ward or outside having a smoke with the desperadoes, it is pretty much this, or Subway.

In addition to the space itself, another restorative feature here is the noticeboard onto which people pin prayers of thanks and pleas for divine assistance. It's an instructive but bittersweet read. Not only are there those worse off than you, but also those of simpler and more loving disposition facing sterner odds in crueller battles. I crave salvation, but it seems I must first wade through shame.

'Please watch over my father and make sure he is safe . . .'

'Please help our family through this difficult time . . . watch over my dad and give him the strength to live through me.'

I am embarrassed. It would never occur to me to say these things, and so I read them out loud. Borrowed emotions, no less true for the lending. I feel better, if reacquainted with a lake of grief I would do anything not to look at.

Another note, 'Hear my plea for sanity . . .'

That I recognize.

In a few hours he's back on the ward, conscious and happy. The incision on his thigh through which they have woven microsurgical magic seems impossibly small. They have also, for good measure, removed the giant growth from his toe. The foot looks almost normal. Still a foot that has seen close to a century of action, but less like something designed by H. R. Giger – a hobbit's nightmare.

He is on morphine, which has the subtle side effect of making him more left-wing. He watches a programme on his bedside TV about George Bernard Shaw and can't stop talking about it. He shows me a profile of a Labour MP in the paper and says that she seems nice. This is not the normal run of things.

He hovers in a kind of dream state common to the opiated. This combines with another of the drug's celebrated side effects, constipation, producing a ten-minute anecdote about whether he has taken a shit.

'In the end it was a dream,' he reveals, eventually.

I am lost for words at the extent and detail of this non-story.

'I'm telling you this,' he says, earnestly, 'so you can put it in a screenplay.'

It has been nearly a decade since I worked on a successful film. Still, his grasp of the market seems as firm as his bowels.

Marginal Gains

For a man who treasures quiet, hospital is hard. The endless beeps, unanswered alarms, the yells of dementia and the cries of lucid need. It accumulates. He can't sleep. Neither can Mum, which is making her edgy. We are all nagged by the same question.

When is he coming home?

Post-op and without any other issues arising, his recovery becomes a matter for the hospital physios. They will determine if he is well enough to be discharged. Their remit to rehome seems extensive and urgent, like military doctors compelled to countenance unready conscripts at the end of a war. You'll do.

Though he could probably be killed by a well-kicked football, Dad is quickly passed as 'medically fit'. Until last year a system of convalescent homes had helped my parents' friends to bridge the gap from hospital to home, but these are closed now. Dismantled by the state.

I have been here before. If you do not go into bat over this they will pronounce your relative fit with a congratulatory smile, but the effect is more like opening a silver dish to reveal some roadkill. What, you wonder, am I supposed to do with that?

The sick person, hitherto attended by a retinue of experts and a rough militia of dispassionate love, is now yours again. To prevent this vulnerable and demanding man landing with too great a thud on his frail and reflexively accommodating wife and near-psychotic younger son, the latter must do some lobbying. Ironically, this requires appearing even less stable than I actually am.

Job number one here is to spell out the indisputable truth of our equation. If he comes home and relies on her, they will both end up in here.

'Do you live at home?' will be the next question to me, and it is a tough one to answer. Yes, but I need all the help I can get, is one way of looking at it. I can't be there all the time, is what I say. Both are true.

To get some sense of what life will be like at home, there are two things to establish. Can he go to the toilet on his own and can he use stairs? It would be a mistake to take these for simple matters. The truth of both is wildly subjective. It would be simpler to run a murder inquiry.

First witness is my father.

'Can you go to the toilet?'

He shrugs. I ask the nurses.

'Has he been to the toilet?'

The ward sister, whose busy demeanour belies a willingness to answer any question, is sadly absent. No one here now has been here when it's happened. His movements then are either a rumour or a rarity. Somewhere between the yeti and a harvest moon. I wait then, like a wildlife cameraman, for nature to take its course.

The Old Man's bowel awakens, and he summons a bedpan.

'So you don't go the toilet, then, in the sense of getting up and going there?'

He shrugs again.

'I might fall over.'

Having established this baseline I find the physios and we set 'getting to the toilet' as a stated goal. I know my dad like a trainer knows his elephant. If he doesn't believe he can do it then he just won't go. A one-off performance for the physios does not equal mobility. The house is like a theatre, we can't afford to book him unless it is for multiple shows.

A hospital admission, I have learnt, leads to a rapid de-skilling on all sides. A haemorrhaging of tolerance and ability in both the cared for and the caring. It makes for messy reunions. It is not the technical skills that desert us, one can still do the things, but the emotional framework that sustains the actions. That's what suffers. This perhaps is what we really mean by coping.

Over time and in a crisis, what you take for normality is in fact a persistent crescendo. Each instrument of your being is played so hard and altogether that to pick any of it up again once you've stopped seems daunting. Impossible even. You feel like a dog with a cello. Sometimes you don't know what you're carrying until you collapse.

For every skill we drop, Dad surrenders another, hospital sustaining him from a prone position. Help available here at the touch of a button. The ability to walk, and any measure of self-reliance, recede entwined as the days go by.

14 January 2018

After two weeks of freedom, Mum is still sleepless, anxious and confused. But she is clear enough about one thing. She can't cope with what she imagines the future will consist of. I promise she won't have to, but, as I keep saying, we'll have to get help. She tightly acquiesces to that, which means she doesn't agree at all, but will suffer it.

'I didn't sign up for this,' she says, again. Plenty of that going around.

'People in the house', as they call it, is an oft-stated fear, but it's that or homes for one or both. And I am here in the meantime, of course, as long as it takes, whatever it takes, and perhaps forever.

Having set the physical parameters for Dad's return, we must now establish the social framework. We are familiar from past admissions with 'Urgent Care', the local government/ NHS hybrid A-Team who see to a paroled patient's needs until they either suddenly learn to tap-dance, die, or need more abiding cover.

This system, which brings a motley, barely scheduled but fundamentally kind and necessary crew of underpaid heroes to your door, lasts for up to six weeks. Or at least it used to. After that, depending on your finances and fitness, it's down to you. It bears mentioning that everyone throughout the assessment process reassures us that we will not be left alone.

What complicates matters is that my father will say anything to get home, including 'my wife looks after me' (true in part, but not sustainable), and 'my son lives with us' (massive silent scream). And, one of his stone-cold classics, 'X [which could be me, Mum or anyone not present whose compliance is attached to some future goal] doesn't mind.' Here, perhaps, is a Post-it note on the fridge to all mankind:

Just because someone does a thing quietly, that does not mean they do not mind.

Or that a thing done once can or should be done forever.

I am anxious not to replicate the traumas of the past, if only for my own sake. I still bear guilt from his last long hospital admission. He was desperate to come home but in no shape to do so. The hospital judged him fit, Mum and I felt differently. A consultant had told him he could go home. After I had lobbied the physios, they agreed, unilaterally I suspect, to keep him two more days.

He was ready to go when I told him he couldn't, and he sobbed. In that moment it was as though he was the child and I the parent. I felt cold and selfish, but it was the right thing to do at the time. I understand now that what's right can still feel awful. Trying to feel good *and* function can break you. Part of us needs to shut down in order to get through. The part that wants everything to be 'all right'.

A City Frieze

Confident the physio's targets are in line with our abilities, and that the dissonant factions of the hospital and our family are on the same page, I can flee for the weekend. A good friend has gone on holiday and lent me their apartment in London. I am dizzy with anticipation, but when I reach the city all I have is dizziness. The streets, the people, even the adverts breed dislocation, and a strange distress. It is not until I get into the flat and sit down that I feel, for the first time in a long time, the extraordinary truth of being alone.

With no one to call out, no one to tend to and absolutely no appointments, something inside me dissolves. This becomes almost literal when I take a bath with the radio on and lie there, unable and unwilling to move, for nearly two hours. Then sleep, un-drugged, for eight, waking just once in the belief that someone has called my name, then recalling where I am and where I'm not, and falling back to sleep again.

Ironically, perhaps, it is a feeling I can only equate with coming out of hospital having been a long-term patient myself, or home after months of work abroad. A sense that life is suddenly different, but with no idea quite what to do.

19 January 2018

I have breakfast with a friend I haven't seen for months. The cafe is playing a song I love but haven't heard for years. Confidence fills me as I relay the pressures of the recent past. It is powerful to have a fresh witness, to testify to one who has not suffered updates all along. To share the whole, and to be heard.

'It sounds like you're doing all right,' he says.

Perhaps. I feel reborn. I may not know where I am going, but I am starting to remember who I was and what I am.

Then I get a text from my brother.

They will let Dad out tomorrow. Can I come home? Of course. But no sooner have I replied than I am claimed by anger and depression. Whatever was reborn seems suddenly premature. It was fun, but the old world is winning and feels worse for the taste of respite. Now I know what life *could* be.

I go for a drink, but can't think of anything else but what is coming or shake the sense of how I really feel. Lost, and drawn back into a situation I don't know if I can endure. Old resentments rise like an undigested meal, so tangible now that I am also surprised and ashamed. What is all this . . . feeling? What is it *for*? I suspect that this isn't about my father, but everybody, everything. Including, and perhaps especially, me.

Contrary to folk idioms, tomorrow comes.

PART THREE

Get Back

I head towards my family with foreboding. There is something robotic in how I navigate the hospital, the staff and my father, like the Terminator called home for the weekend.

My brother, whose empathy is deep but available only on an occasional basis, senses this as we help the Old Man home and into the house. He gives me a knowing look. I've had some good trips back from the hospital before, full of hope, buoyed myself by the relief in Dad's eyes as soon as we are in the taxi. This isn't one of them. Something good, or merely tolerant, in me has gone.

*

With Dad back in his chair and Mum making the best of it, Liam, the council care coordinator, arrives and we sit in the kitchen and discuss what to do. Liam unpacks ring binders, laminated sheets and handouts and spreads them before him in a defensive informational fan, like a blackjack dealer. Dad will get two visits, he says. One in the morning, to help him up and into the shower and get him dressed. One in the evening to do the reverse. This is as it was when he was last in need.

We know how it goes. I also know the answer to the next question, but I ask it anyway.

'What time will they come?'

'We do our best,' shrugs Liam. 'But it's not a time pacific service.'

Sadly for me, the mild and unacknowledged misuse of language is something that tweaks my weakest nerve, and today I am already borderline postal. The substitution of 'pacific' for 'specific' is a particularly troubling one. I am convinced that people prone to this are on some level testing you, to see if you say something about it. As Pacific Liam is holding all the cards here, laminated and otherwise, I manage not to react. But he keeps pushing me.

'We can't offer pacific slots.'

God help me. I am more bothered by the language than the vagaries of the system. I accept the institutional shortcomings and am genuinely grateful that anyone comes at all. I don't have time to dwell on my own largesse since more troubling information is coming. Liam asks if my dad still has savings and owns the house. He does.

'Then in two weeks you'll need to find your own care, if he still needs it.'

'We'll need it,' I confirm.

Liam pushes leaflets towards me. Cashing me out of the game.

'I thought it was seven weeks?'

'No. Two.'

'Last year it was seven.'

'Now it's two,' says Liam, adding, 'You won't be left alone.'

I tell Mum and Dad. The pressing detail for them is that people will now come to the house at a range of non-specified times. I say, 'They can't be pacific,' a few times and we wrangle the matter into a joke. But Mum is serious.

'How will I know when to be ready?'

'You won't need to be ready,' I say. 'They're coming so you don't have to do things. And I'm here.'

'I won't know when to get up,' she protests. 'And I still don't get much sleep.'

That night a carer comes who smells so densely of cigarettes that, as a child of smokier times, I find it reassuring. Beyond the tobacco the scent of compassion is stronger. They work the city silently, these smoky saviours, stepping out of tiny cars just as you were losing hope. Mum gives him a nickname, 'Puffing Billy'. And he is, like my father, weaker for his habit. It takes them a while to get up the stairs together. Thus Dad, 'stair fit', allegedly, heaves himself along the double banisters like some ancient gymnast, with me behind and Billy ahead.

Billy, it turns out, has COPD as well. We make quite the team. We stop along the way like mountaineers, pitching base camps. Regrouping. Forging on. What Billy lacks in lung he brings in heart and he is soon a favourite on the roster. Not that there is a roster. You take whatever and whoever comes.

Tears for Fears

I wake abruptly at 4 a.m. Not to some external stimulus but to a feeling of such pure and primal grief that it is like something standing on your stomach. Several things. Age-old infants of despair, rousing me to feed them. The chemical solution is inches away. But I don't want to drug myself back to sleep any more; I want to get beyond this. So I get up and sit in a chair to see where it takes me. Come, sadness, do your thing. A conglomerate sorrow, my life's savings, in a sense, floods through me.

I know things are bad at 4.20 because I have a photograph that shows the time. Tears are surpassed by great ectoplasmic trails of phlegm. All this cascades onto the pale grey of my tracksuit bottoms until it appears I have joined the roll call of incontinence and spilled drinks. I am upset, but also fascinated by the sheer amount of fluid available for this. It is for that, I think, I take a picture on my phone of the stain. I tell myself this act of observation means I am not yet insane, terminally shaken or irretrievably stirred. These woes that call me to think them through for the thousandth time are being watched. If that slender but sane observer in me can record things, then perhaps they have purpose. The sad, insatiable children recede, off my chest and out of my mind. They gather in the shadows as if awaiting some verdict. Free of these galling spirits, perhaps I can fashion a conclusion.

Since there is nothing to be done about what has happened, there are no worthwhile thoughts to give it. No power and no plans. I am in a negotiation with myself.

You feel terrible. OK, I hear you. What's next?

My friend was right back in December. I should write more of this down. Or wait to get locked up.

In daylight I can make no sense of what happened in the dark. Why last night and not some other, what is all this inner drama for? There seems no logic to these feelings, but I know that they were so. I have the pictures, after all, theme park souvenirs from some demented ride. Perhaps love and despair have something in common. Neither will be told exactly where to go. With my internal dialogue in such comprehensive chaos I turn myself over to the radio.

It would be wrong not to salute the healing role of music in this uncertain journey. I have found as I have got older that pop music, once the driving force of my existence, a love affair begun within these very walls, is rife with truly terrible advice. In the light of this I have given up my radio to a classical station which, this particular morning, plays a song from the year 1530. Infused with a sense of the human continuum in a way that protestations of adolescent problems from the 1980s can no longer provide, I march downstairs, admit the morning carer and set to breakfast renewed.

'You show those eggs who's boss,' says Mum as she watches. Sometimes all we need is a witness and a tune.

22 January 2018

If today were a film we might run these scenes as montage. Carer in, Dad up, me in front of laptop as I throw down breakfast. The race is on. While the pros are here, I am highly motivated. And slightly mental. If we can get continuing care in place, then I can get out of here. For what and to where is not the issue. For now I have a plan. After so long with what seemed like so little, this is enough. I recall I am alive. Let's go.

As I wash up, I talk to this morning's carer about how difficult I have found things and she opens up about her own family. A lot comes out; it takes twenty minutes of Dad's allocated hour. She says she finds it easier to treat strangers with dementia than she did to care for her own mum. I hear that one.

The district nurses come and check Dad's progress and reassure him that being out of hospital does not mean he has slipped from medical view. As they leave, they ask if there is anything else they can do for him.

'Stay with me all day,' he says in an entreating voice I never hear directly.

The nurses say, 'Ah,' and hold his hand.

I suppress a giant 'Fuck you.'

I call Liam. He remains rigidly pacific about the two-week deadline, 'but we won't leave you on your own'. He gives the name of an agency he recommends, which is something. Care is a sellers' market, aggressively so. Too many needing and not enough supply. Half-decent agencies run at capacity. Getting a callback from anyone in the ideal bullseye of the Harold Shipman to not-giving-a-shit matrix becomes a minor triumph. Even if they have the availability, they must come and assess us, and us them. It takes time and a certain level of determination. You are in effect giving up your parents for adoption.

After Dad's heart attacks last year, I dissolved days on the Care Quality Commission website (a kind of high-stakes Tripadvisor for the elderly), so I know the game and which local firms are worth speaking to. I work the phone all morning. Two weeks is no time in which to sort things out.

I email a charity about the statutory guidelines for this. The rules are impenetrable online. How this works from an elderly perspective if you don't have vengeful, persuasive offspring with time on their hands, I can't imagine.

I place an advert on a specialist website asking for a dedicated, non-agency person. We attach a key safe to the wall so that carers can come and go without rousing the natives. This is a big step. Anxieties over security and assertions of independence had blocked this game-changing adaptation in the past, perhaps rightly. Now it's done. It is hard when things get harder but also a relief when certain needs become non-negotiable. Pain saves debate.

By the end of the day there are emails and phone messages from me across the county and beyond. For the first time in a long time I feel like I might have got something done. An effect. I can also see that all my notes, records and recollections might add up to something, a story of sorts. In real terms, nothing has happened yet, but the world is turning and I am not so nauseous any more.

23 January 2018

In the morning there is an email from the charity Age UK which is clearer than anything I have received in hospital or from the council. But it is not news I especially want.

What is known locally as Urgent Care is more widely described as Intermediate Care, if I am reading my fact sheets correctly. 'Intermediate Care can be misunderstood,' explains the charity, 'so it is important to know it is *not* a period of free care that you are always entitled to following a stay in hospital.'

Liam is right. They can call it how they see it. What Intermediate Care is about, apparently, is 'potential for further improvement'. Hence the variable margins. The council carers are here 'to help you reach your goals'. But our goals, I suspect, are not in alignment. I wonder sometimes if Dad has any goals at all.

24 January 2018

Time to address the transport and logistics situation. I need a bike. My sister has a knack of reclaiming hers when I need it most, which has left me trudging to her house to fetch it, a spectacle which reliably summons rain. And then it still collapses. I call my brother, consistently the most financially fluid of us, and he gives me the money for a bicycle of my own.

I bus into town where there are two-wheeled winter sale bargains aplenty, and ride happily home. I could be sixteen again. When I reach the house, I ride past and on around the neighbourhood until it gets dark. This being January, that doesn't take long, but it feels good.

The carers continue to come, dependably erratic but consistently kind. They are also, by the demographics of our household, the shock troops of modernity. Diverse and festooned with contemporary accessories. 'I couldn't stop looking at it!' says Mum of one's nose-piercing. It's as though characters from their television have walked directly into the room.

25 January 2018

I get an encouraging email from my friend Ron who lives abroad and knows a lot about energy:

In electricity there is a term: load-shedding. Required to keep the power supply constant, in some way. A technical thing. I hope for some equivalent for you.

He is right. I go to London, shed that load a little, write and reflect and confess.

The Mighty Fall

28 January 2018

In my brief absence my benign, or perhaps lacklustre, regime has been replaced by a surveillance-gathering operation run by the unlikely but effective partnership of my deaf mum and suspicious sister. On the train home I get an email from her outlining in minute detail what has taken place in the forty-eight hours since I left. It is long but instructive. Perspective is important in this. You need other voices. More, perhaps, than what they say. My sister reports on my father's latest visit from the district nurse:

We heard her tell him he needed to 'be honest about his diet' to aid recovery, eat proteins etc. I asked what we could do to help, she emphasised diet, I asked about biscuits in night and she said no, and not alcohol either . . . not while the infection is still there. She didn't like the look of his foot.

No one, unless they worked in special effects make-up, would like the look of his foot. He has not been healing as the hospital hoped, and the Scotch and shortbread will not be helping. This is an old story, though, an almost functional dysfunction. More worrying is what she writes about Mum.

Mum says she 'cannot cope', can't see her friends 'while I am like this'. And on a trip to Boots couldn't tell a display of bottled water from the items she had just bought.

This is harder to take, but there is a chance that Mum's decline could be down to her meds. I certainly hope so.

Another salient detail from my sister is that she has opened a box that was too large for our folks to manage and discovered dozens of pairs of socks from Amazon inside. If Dad is back with Bezos then something deep within the man himself is stirring. He is coming back online.

29 January 2018

I call the GP, who agrees Mum can stop taking mirtazapine in advance of her review appointment later in the week. She is too new to the drug to go into withdrawal, they say. On balance the medication seems to have made her worse, or she is becoming worse in a way that the medication cannot help.

'Thank God,' she says when I tell her she can stop taking it.

'How are you coping?' I ask.

'Fine.'

'That's not what you told your daughter, is it?'

She raises an immense scowl at this cross-examination. But if we aren't the cops then there are none and chaos reigns.

'If you want our help then you need to get your story straight. We can't act on one thing if you're telling someone else another.'

Consistency may have long since fled the scene, and Mum shuffles away in a world of her own, but I can't build a case for change with so much contradictory testimony. Or at least a case that I can live with and act on. And there must be action, since now the world is calling.

I'm offered a couple of weeks' work in London. Temporary teaching. White-collar, gig-economy stuff; take it or leave it. The pay isn't much and would be wiped out by the cost of commuting, so I would need to stay up there. But this isn't about money, this is about me without them and them without me, a chance to see if that can be sustained. By any of us.

A photographer friend of mine decamps from London to Africa for the winter to save money and follow the sun, so his flat is available. He just needs the bills paid and plants watered. I want it, and fate wants it too. I should go. Pacific Liam's recommended care company have availability to tend to Dad morning and evening and are coming for a meeting.

This might all work out.

I make tea and go to John's to watch television.

*

Five minutes into the evening football my mobile rings. It's Mum, telling me to come home.

'He's fallen over.'

Experience has removed 'why?' and 'how?' from my instinctive vocabulary. So home I go, on my new bike, just a means to an end now. The January night, dark and cold as a cellar, reaches under my collar and on into my bones.

A kind of tableau confronts me indoors. A graphic set piece, dense with symbols and players.

Dad lies sprawled on the landing. Comfortable, he says, but

somewhat crazed-looking. The man from next door, a gallant figure who, with his wife, provides a neighbourly safety net I would not want to work without, is scrubbing blood off the stair carpet.

Tonight's carer, a stranger to us, as is often the way, is shuffling about near my dad while on the phone to her supervisors.

'I can't pick him up and I can't go upstairs behind him and he just . . . fell,' she explains, somewhat coldly. But I know she is right. The risk of a carer being taken out as collateral in a stair fall is too great. The ones who will help him upstairs are transgressive, rule-breakingly generous. This, then, is where the rubber of the hospital's 'stair fit' assessment meets the hard road of our reality, and explodes.

Mum meanwhile is on the phone to III, the non-urgent emergency service. She's making the random affirmative noises she makes when she can't hear you. I take the phone. Dad will bleed in a stiff breeze, so things likely aren't quite as bad as they appear.

We are on hold. I notice that the bloody stair where he slipped is the same one our long-dead cat would claw at years ago. Dad took her to be put down and spoke then of foreseeing his own end. Now here we are. Same staircase, different demise.

The neighbour and I get Dad to his feet and into his bedroom. The neighbour goes home. Cold-but-correct carer goes on to their next call. Then it's just me and the Old Man and the voice on the phone.

The operator asks questions which I relay to my father. He answers with a series of untruths he thinks will keep him out of hospital. Sometimes I think he's lost the plot, but when it comes to it he can still master the game.

You can intercede in this stuff and have an ambulance come (which can take hours, if they're not on a blue light), or you can relay the self-effacing fibs that belie the severity of the situation and spin the wheel at home. I choose the latter. He deserves a break. He's only been back here for eight days. He seems OK, ish. And I don't want to wait around any more than he does. Things might get worse, but sometimes worse is what you wish for. So we reassure the earthly powers we need no intervention tonight, hang up the phone and consign ourselves to forces unknown.

30 January 2018

In the morning he feels better, he says, but it will be his last time upstairs. Farewell to his bedroom of forty-two years. Adieu to the shower. As I shepherd him down the stairs with the morning carer I tread over the bloodstained cat step and wonder when my time will come. It's a hereditary thing, morbidity, in every conceivable sense.

Thanks to my sister's long-range radar of paranoia we are prepped for these events. The first tier of the second-hand market in pricey end-of-life accessories is entirely word-of-mouth. My sister likes to talk in the same way as sharks like to keep moving; she knows a lot of people, and her connection to those with serious illnesses is enough to suggest causality. Some years back the mother of a friend of hers died and her motorized hospital-style bed became available. My sister bought it and stashed it in the spare bedroom – a feat only accomplished by her friend removing a window here to make space for the manoeuvre. These are heavy things. At the time I wasn't paying much attention. Now all our problems have coalesced into one pulsing mass of challenges we laughingly call life.

I must get the bed downstairs and make a bedroom in the back room I had been using as retreat-cum-office. As I clear my desk I am reminded that none of this can last. I have lost this space, another island outpost of self, to the rising tide of reality. But if the tearful scenes and inner torment have taught me anything, it's that the self is a notional thing. The real problem, the tangible hiccup in the here and now, is that I have no idea how you remove a UPVC window.

I am rescued by John who is a genius for this stuff and arrives tooled up to assist. By assist I mean do more or less everything. It takes less than an hour, thanks to his prowess with an electric screwdriver, to remove the double banisters the occupational therapy team have fitted, and get the bed, which is like a small car, downstairs. No window removal necessary.

While he gets the banisters back up, I redistribute the old furniture and build a bedroom in the space once reserved for celebratory dinners and the Pharaonic clutter of long lives. Candlesticks, cutlery, doilies and dust.

If I say so myself, the room looks amazing. Or perhaps I'm just tired. I lie on the bed and raise myself up and down as though I'm in *The Exorcist*. This is sensational. Why wait until you're old to get this stuff? I am annoyed that I haven't been sleeping in this one until now. Mum catches me at it and likes what she sees. She takes a turn and is in agreement. This is now the best room in the house.

I take a picture and send it to my siblings. An unfamiliar sensation is returning, normally felt before a fall. Pride. Take that, proverbial wisdom. As ever, some cosmic force is listening, forming a vengeful smile.

You Get What You Need

I awake with the peculiar sense of freedom known only to those with unobstructed access to a bathroom. I take my time, then fetch Dad a tea.

His new room faces south. Morning light streams into it, even in this dingy season. To me it looks amazing. Dad's face, though, speaks to some inner issue, beyond the whims of weather or interior design. How does he feel?

'Not so good, son. Not so good.'

Confusingly for those of us close to him, this is a phrase that is used for everything from near death to mild discomfort. Personally, selfishly, I am annoyed that he doesn't seem as pleased as I am about the room. The sense that my efforts are unrecognized might be underwriting part of what happens next.

A carer comes. She asks what she should do. I am near enough to hear Dad say to her that he won't get up to brush his teeth. That he now must be tended to lying down, as if in hospital. This, in my sister's parlance, is a slippery slope, and Dad, it seems, has got his skis on. I go into the room.

'You have to at least try and get up,' I say.

He won't look at me. It is hard to convey the conflict between the instinctive sympathy one feels with a frail, elderly person, and the parallel wave of resentment when it seems that person is wilfully engaging in a series of decisions that rest on the assumption that – regardless of consequence or cost to those around – the world will bend to their will, or the apparent lack thereof.

I try and lay it out calmly. I feel anything but. One must be careful. Throw on all the childhood psycho-baggage, and the camel's back of care collapses. The sense of rectitude rises when you have absolute power over those who once had it over you. I don't need righteous anger, I have enough of the regular kind. I get a grip, breathe, spell it out s-l-o-w-l-y:

'Two nights ago we didn't go to hospital because you swore you didn't need to go to hospital. Now you want the house, which we spent yesterday rebuilding to further accommodate you, to work more like a hospital. Since you share it and depend on the wellness of an eighty-nine-year-old woman whose own health, mental and physical, is negatively impacted by the decline in yours and the compromises and pressures on how we live as a result, that isn't gonna work. You have to *try* and get out of bed. This bed that will elevate you to make that easier than ever before. If you need more care than this . . . then you have to go somewhere that can be supplied. That would be a care home.'

It's *Rocky* in reverse. The fitter, younger fighter fights to train the trainer. This is my most desperate and I hope persuasive move to get him back in the ring. He's not messing about, though. He goes for the big one.

'Then I want to die.'

Is this what it comes down to? Nine decades on the planet and you want to check out rather than try to stand up? I don't even know what's going on inside of me, let alone him. I do know, though, that the carer is going about her business, clearing up the catheter clutter as we carry on.

I say I'm sorry. She gives me a look which says, or I interpret as: she's seen and heard all this before. I am reassured that this dialogue, which feels extreme, might in fact be rather normal. Nevertheless, I ask her to give us a minute, which she does.

Again, he says –

'I want to die.'

There is a symbiotic moment of possibility here since there is a part of me, in this raging instant, which would happily assist him.

I wonder if that is how these things happen. This is how you make the papers. One of those stories that seem distant and unfathomable, until you are suddenly inside them. Just a few decisions from infamy.

He and I know well enough now why there was a stash of temazepam in his wardrobe and some Bacardi. This was his exit strategy. My mother and sister speak of hoarding and of alcoholism, but they have not done the maths here. Nor have I ever shared the conversation Dad and I had long ago about this outcome. I think I said that if it came to it, and he was sure, then I would help him. Now what I say instead is –

'Do it, then. The drugs are upstairs. Get yourself up there and I'll give you a hand.'

What I don't add to this is that my brother and I have taken so much temazepam in the last year, you would be hard pressed to assemble an overdose from the remainder. A hell of a nap, but nothing longer. Even if we had reached a euthanistic consensus amicably, we lack the goods to pull it off.

He doesn't counter, which makes things worse. I end on a kind of threat.

'You can lie there and end up somewhere else, or you can try and do more and stay here.'

Like all threats one ought to be able to back it up, but I don't even know who I am in this any more. I go to lie down, but not before Mum trundles past half-naked on the landing.

'Everything all right?' she asks cheerfully.

'Oh yeah,' I answer, feeling as bad as I ever felt in my life, adding –

'It's all good.'

'Good,' she says, which means she might have heard me.

This is the least of anyone's worries. Managing contingent fictions is how we run this house. Sometimes the truth is as much use as staring into the sun.

Lying down is impossible. You may as well try and nap in flames. I call my brother. Not something I am wont to do at 8 a.m. unless something is up. He senses this, and hears me out patiently as I outline the morning in the way one might describe an assailant. Though I don't know if I am the perpetrator or the victim here.

Something in me, something in our family structure and recent and ancient pasts, makes me desperate to be able to handle all this, to be the one that makes things work. To admit to my brother, my *older* brother, that I can't, is like both needing and resenting the police. That I am out of moves here and struggling to go on, is quite a thing. All exacerbated perhaps by the fact these are the apparent qualities, or perceived lack thereof, that I find so troubling in my father. This will be a fun week in therapy, if I can get there.

For now there is nowhere to hide. Especially not your childhood bedroom. I must go downstairs and see what's what before Mum gets there and gets upset or confused or both. And maybe I need to apologize. Someone does.

When I get to the kitchen Dad is at the table, eating. The carer is leaving. Has he got up to prove me wrong or right? Has he found the strength or was he hiding it? Suddenly I am full of the sadness of it all, and the shame. I sit next to him as he clanks through his porridge, stabbing his spoon against the bowl.

I take his hand.

'I am sorry,' I say. 'I don't know what else to do here.'

'It's OK,' he tells me.

And then I'm crying, again.

'I never saw you much when I was a kid and I guess I want something now, some example to hang on to. Something I can use and remember. I don't know who or how to be in all this.'

I'm gesturing at the house, but I mean the world.

'This is our last chance. Let's not fuck it up.'

Old Lady Land

I still want out. Eight days before I'm due to start work, and with the morning behind us, we sit politely like normal people who haven't just been threatening murder-suicide, and meet one of the managers from the care company.

This firm was Pacific Liam's hot tip. The manager is lovely and so by inference must her legions be. What else can you go on? Mum and Dad acquiesce politely to a future of continued care. And that is not nothing. 'People in the house' twice a day, perhaps forever. You wouldn't have sold that here a few weeks ago.

'Look,' I say to Mum when we have a moment. 'It can't go on for long, can it?'

By this we mean how long does he have, and who are we to shape that time to fit our own desires? This is what we tell ourselves in quieter times.

1 February 2018

Dad rises without complaint, assisted by the carer. My sister drives Mum to the shops. When she does come back having bought herself something to wear, Mum is beside herself, overjoyed.

'I am in old lady land now,' she announces, wielding a pair of trousers in the manner of one planting a flag into some hitherto unknown country. 'No more zips. Just these elastic waists.'

A district nurse comes and winces at my father's toe, as is the way with those new to it.

'I don't like how this looks,' she says. 'And I can smell it.'

She takes pictures of the unhealed and festering hole, like a crime scene or some injured celebrity, and we up Dad's antibiotics. He clanks off into the bathroom on his frame. I ask the nurse what will happen if the infection doesn't shift. She says that won't be her decision. Hospital, then? Maybe. I am almost sad about that. I had dared to think this could work at home, if he and I tried, and with help from the professionals. The nurse leaves.

'I have opened my bowels,' Dad announces from the bathroom.

There is no corner of the house where you could not have known. He has been constipated since hospital and now this has passed. One grim internal season lurching into another. I feel like Robert Duvall praising the smell of napalm, but this is good news.

Interior Worlds

If I am ever going to get anything done, I need a desk. This means a trip to town. First, I head to my sister's and take a bath. I miss baths. I do this infrequently enough to forget that for a person of my height, my sister's bath is just a deep bidet. I curl up inside until it gets cold. Then I go to IKEA.

For a number of reasons, chiefly a profound disposition for letting other people take care of things, I have only been here once in the twenty-odd years since it came to our shores. I think I was twenty-six last time, one of my wife's early attempts to lure me into maturity, and I hated it then. Coming back at almost fifty is a real kick in the psychological balls.

I have no clue how it works. I have seen that people riot for this stuff, but I feel like I have fallen from space.

I am scurrying and startled and occasionally stunned still, like that film about the pig in the city. Wishing some fellow farmyard thing would help me out.

In time, hours, it seems, I find a 'desk', in fact a chic, spindly table, named almost entirely out of consonants. I somehow pay for it. In a final twist of the life-comparison knife, this place also hates you if you don't have a car. I haul my self-assembly SKTNA, or whatever it's called, through the multi-level car park like a dwarf in some mythic saga, dragging a sacred weapon it can barely wield from hell. Hiding from traffic until I reach the unfashionable pavement, just me and RKNHA and the litter in the breeze. I wait for a taxi and feel oddly at peace.

Cars full of families and furniture trundle past us all the while. I had an arrogant, defensive streak as a teenager growing up here and didn't want to be like the others. Mission accomplished. Now look upon me from your hybrids and despair, squares. A strange pride fills me as I stuff LNHGI into a cab.

In an Ideal World

My brother has taken Mum to the doctor, who has put her on amitriptyline, a drug she used some years ago. The results are near instantaneous. She sleeps, rises rested and seems to look about her fearlessly again.

I'm dubious about long-term psychiatric medication, but this is a startling turnaround. And she is happy. She keeps saying so. With each proclamation the margins of my grief recede.

'You have to get out of here,' my brother tells me. 'It's not healthy.'

'I'm going, I've got some work.'

I want him to look worried since this is surely major news. How will they cope without me? But he doesn't.

'Good,' he says.

Plumbers come again to see if they can stop the heating sounding like a locomotive. One takes me aside and says the whole system is so old they can't entirely solve the problem without replacing everything. I have heard this before about my father. Stay still long enough and you become the space that surrounds you.

In an Ideal World

I love the new carers. Three seem especially careful and kind. Again I find myself thinking that this might all work smoothly from now on. Dad rattles this blissful fantasy by sending one away for coming 'too early'. The carer acquiesces and comes back later, which, given the zero-hours, no-time-for-transit nature of their employment, will have cost him money. I suggest to Dad that if you mess the good people around then the good people will go. If we weren't wrapped in the DNA chain I might have fled myself by now. I think this but don't say it, in case he says, 'where to?' I still can't answer that. It's mid February. Twelve months since I first came home, and I think with all this assistance I can see a way out, if not a destination.

Just as things are looking up, the council close the road that leads to our house overnight for the next month. How will the carers get here? What if it snows? 'A permit system is in operation', promise the council, who are presently turning off streetlights to save money. No one is convinced.

'We might be stranded.'

'Fear will finish you off sooner than starvation,' I suggest.

This is supposed to be encouraging. But the elders are a tough crowd, you never quite know how things land. And with such vague but threatening reassurance ringing in their ears – if they even heard me – I slip away to London and to work.

15 February 2018

As ever, there is no escape from my sister's emails. Dad is watching Westerns and not moving, she informs me. Mum, still improving, tells her she 'would like the house back', which means the spare and otherwise unused room in which Dad sleeps. None of this is actionable. These are standard laments. We pass them between us dutifully and do nothing. We are the results in part of what our loved ones get around to or away with.

My sister says that she and Mum had been out and came back to find Dad microwaving some soup. *He promptly sat down and asked mum to finish it,* she writes, *and then swore at me for saying he was doing well and [asking] what would have happened if we'd got home 5 mins later?*

My sister's idea of a benign inquiry could provoke a papal candidate to profanity, but she is onto something here. This is Dad at his most dissembling. Her report continues:

He said 'in an ideal world I should be in bed all day'!!

I tell her to tell him that if he aspires to be in bed all day there are places where that can happen. The house with Mum isn't one of them.

It is so hot, she goes on, that walking through the door there, *is like stepping off a plane in Alicante.*

Dad will, I've noticed, leave his frame behind and scale a couple of stairs to reach the thermostat if it is on anything less than maximum. This revival is enabled by his fundamental faith that it is always freezing. This is such a constant source of aggravation that it is almost a relief when, days later, everything genuinely freezes, and it snows.

27 February 2018

My sister keeps the folks supplied as the country battles through arctic weather. The carers make it to the house too. No mean achievement, given the depth of the snow and the incline of the road. One morning they don't, and Mum gets Dad up alone.

'Like dressing a baby,' she reflects over the phone, 'but a baby's skin is softer.' Imagination and pragmatism are as ever her chief allies when confronting the unknown. She is equally buoyant about swallowing her new nightly tablet.

'If I'm struggling to get it down,' she tells me, 'I pretend the SS are coming up the stairs.'

Work is good. Students take me at face value, know nothing of my past or wider present and for a few hours a day I can assert competence, be heard and get paid. I feel like a participant in the world instead of a passenger, even as I slump down on the Tube afterwards. In the evenings I write up the notes I've made into more coherent pages. I read back over our recent past and smile. The pleasures of perspective and the relief of solitude. But this is all fleeting. I am on borrowed time in borrowed spaces.

2 March 2018

This tenuous, temporary contract with the capital is physicalized when I visit my old belongings in a storage unit out in the badlands where London edges into Essex. Snow is falling through its broken glass roof. I stare at box after box of I don't know what. The place is so cold that burning everything I own seems physically wise and psychologically desirable, but really I have to get all this back to where I once belonged.

This hurts, inside and out, but it is all my own handiwork. I bite my tongue and get to it. I think of a sailor having surgery before anaesthetic, perhaps because Nelson is a hero of my dad's and I grew up around pictures of men grimacing on gun decks in each other's arms. Odd, that my own martial coping fantasies are set a century before my mum's.

11 March 2018

Back at Old Zero, Dad, bravely, gives up the frame, resuming the walking stick and holding onto furniture routine. A horizontal mountaineer. Things have progressed so far that by Mother's Day both parents are able to get to my brother's for lunch. Happily, this coincides with my retrieving my possessions and moving them back into the house I moved them out of thirty years ago.

We all know this is happening but I'd still rather they didn't see it, or at least weren't in the way or forced to bear witness as I and my nephew ferry decades of crap into the attic, including, I note, books I took with me the first time and still haven't read. Books I thought would make me clever and safe. Books that lost out to impatience, music, people and pubs. I don't imagine there was anything in them that would have stopped any of this from happening, but of course one cannot know.

By the time Mum and Dad get back you wouldn't think anything was different unless you could see into the sagging beams of the attic or my own embarrassed soul. My progress (if that's the word) is as irregular and unpredictable as my parents' recovery, which seems an equally limited term for what they are going through. For now, I'm back again.

Shadows & Dust

15 March 2018

I am upstairs on the phone to a solicitor, reckoning the wreckage of my former life. The billable minutes are clicking towards billable hours when the sounds of parental discord rise from below, like the house band striking up a familiar number in some place you can't believe you still visit. Or the only place that lets you in.

The telephones at my folks', like all else here, are far from modern. A botched network of cordless handsets that seldom make it back to the correct cradle, each with a background hiss that makes everything sound like AM radio. Improving this is somewhere on that list of things to do that I must get around to writing. The solicitor's voice, which I struggle to make sense of on a good day, is relegated even further in my mind as I listen, just as I did as a child, to what my parents are squabbling about. In this case, trousers.

Mum's relationship to ironing is complex, but the essence of today's dispute concerns Dad (who I have never seen iron) asserting that some trousers she has ironed for him (in which he will go nowhere, see no one but her or me, and do nothing but sit down) should have a crease in them.

'You cannot have a crease in cotton trousers,' says Mum.

My father's answer, which comes at a special volume, several notches higher than the one necessary to get Mum to hear you at all, peals through the house –

'I CREATE ONE!'

Given his size and wellness, an utterance of this dimension is an achievement. The dying body is, one presumes, preserving such powers for some desperate and definitive address or plea. Or maybe a sneeze. The scale of window-rattling, primal-scream sneeze that can issue from the elderly frame is quite something. Like a sparrow barking the opening to 'Back in Black'.

The crease creation of which Dad bellows concerns his trouser press, an artefact (now inaccessible upstairs) which speaks to its owner's precision and pride as much as to what I assume (given his military experience) must be unwillingness rather than inability to wield an iron. He is also vulnerable to any full-page advertisement in a Sunday newspaper. If you have ever wondered, 'Who buys *that*?' I have the answer.

Mum can barely lift the iron, the board is taller than she is and yet, unless physically restrained, she will haul it into position and press something, singing as she does so. The singing is a divine reflex, not so much on the technical front – though she can absolutely hold a tune – but for what it signifies, at least to me, now, as in childhood, always mindful of her mood. It takes but a few bars of 'I Could Have Danced All Night', 'The Skater's Waltz' or whatever she has chosen, to disarm all fears of her unhappiness and to marvel at the character on which such joy alights.

As a moaner more than a singer I find this instructive. Those who sing despite their troubles have ever put the rest of us, who sift our pleasures for the next problem, to shame. Might it be, as an old favourite of mine suggests, that happiness is just a state of mind?

As all this drifts through my song-soothed self, the solicitor takes pity and offers to end the call. I concur. I think on my father's sartorial and presentational concerns, on quite how long it will take him and me to get him 'ready' for another day of not much at all.

16 March 2018

When we do go out, the stakes rise and we tense in anticipation. The garments laid out and double-checked the night before. A trip to the doctor's or my brother's, each rendered like a state occasion. I have come to find this a helpful way to think about it. I serve the last royals of an old regime.

In these morning rituals the angle of the sun reveals plumes of perished flesh erupting from Dad's shins and scalp as I pull up his trousers or part his hair. He is crumbling, monumental.

They say dust is dead skin, but it's not until I see this that the constant transaction between who we are, what we're made of, and where we are going becomes quite so clear. On one hand there is revulsion, on another beauty. Look at anything closely enough, long enough and there is wonder to it. Impatience then becomes the enemy of feeling. Love is just attention in the end.

Stuff inside my father forces itself out so often that I take a certain pride in keeping his mosaic of flesh in good condition. Like polishing an old car. It doesn't matter if you don't move it, so long as it shines. I do this so seldom now the carers are here, that I no longer mind. If anything, I feel grounded by it. I fear forgetting how this goes as much as I fear having to do it all the time.

If the light is perfect, you can see the fragments of former skin slow dancing in the air and catch something sublime in it. All my life I have been told I think too much, but at times like this it seems to save me. I wonder if Dad sometimes sees the same way. I believe so. Sometimes it seems the only difference between us is that I have found a way to get these things out, to express them, even if it is to strangers on pages. I send letters to the world like he sent postcards to our family. Face to face is where we fall short. I wish we talked more. Instead, I pull the unsaid about me like a blanket. I have no idea how I would look without it now, or how to put it down.

17 March 2018

With the mortal stakes receding and daylight returning my sister turns her raptor's eye (and maybe deeper need) for action away from the occupants and onto the house itself. Certain issues escape me which are screamingly obvious to her. This time she has her eye on the dust. While I muse over its symbolism, she acts on its dispersal and on its more complex cousin, clutter.

Our parent's cleaner is a benign but lacklustre figure, beset by health issues of her own and often absent. But they like her, and she navigates them. Thus I ask no more of her and do no less, but my sister holds us all to a higher standard, and now launches a series of strikes against the house and its forgotten corners that leave me breathless.

Her conflict with the cleaner puts me in mind of something I learnt on a trip to Bethlehem. The religious factions that hold sway in the church above the site of the manger do battle with each other about who sweeps up, where and why. On occasion the monks fight with brooms and whatever ecclesiastical clutter comes to hand until riot police intervene. By the standards of the region this is tame stuff, and perhaps cathartic, the smaller struggle preventing greater strife. So it goes with the hoover at home. Thus armed, my sister asserts her dominion. Woe to those who might stand in her way.

When cleaning she is frantic yet focused. As if all life depended on it. When we share a mission I am often exhausted at the pace of it, if embarrassed by these strident lessons about what one can accomplish if one tries. My dad hides biscuits, then forgets where these stashes are. My sister's nose for these pockets of calorific self-harm is akin to that of a police dog. She moves through the house like a weather system, talking the whole time. If I weren't caught up in it I might pay to spectate. It's like watching someone breathe underwater.

While she fights the crumbs I can't see, I fight the crap I can. Mountains of DVDs, foothills of old tech and mounds of aimless gadgets are systematically removed. This is very much the tale of our times here. I am working a parallel purge upon my own once-valued possessions, now returned and clearly anything but the sacred relics I had taken them to be. I have a Lutheran revelation. Stuff is just stuff, it turns out. Stuff is not me, nor I it. I am ending one of my lives as my parents balance at the edge of theirs.

18 March 2018

For someone who lives out of a bag, I have way too many books. There is a second-hand stall up the road who will come and collect and the owner is soon on their way back up the hill with a boot-full of beloved tomes. I am relieved that the place is emptying out. This sensation lasts less than a minute before the chemist's envoy appears and drops off a bulging sack of drugs, dressings and catheter equipment. At least the medical supplies won't have to fight for space with five DVDs of *Zulu*, a CD Walkman or a child's thermos flask from 1982.

Heads Up

Despite having grown up in this house and been forced into intimacy with corners, cupboards and bodily crevices I would have preferred to leave undiscovered, there are still things here unknown to me.

This evening, after Dad has been unhitched from his plastic plumbing, connected to the night systems and laid flat by the carer, Mum announces she is heading up to bed. When they are asleep, the place is calm, quiet, beyond the arrhythmic thud and thump of the heating. You can do what you like then. Except I tend to fall asleep as well. First we must gather Mum's stuff before she climbs the stairs.

Unsupervised at this hour she will load herself up with things on every limb: books, a handbag (worn around the neck), tissues, spectacles, glass of milk. Perhaps you have seen the documentary *Free Solo* about the climber who attempts to scale El Capitan without safety ropes? Like that, this is almost unwatchable. She totters upwards, laden with her goods. The disaster is implicit in the exercise – like the kid's game Buckaroo, or repeated acts of bomb disposal. It must eventually go wrong. You either intervene or walk away.

I try and be there for the ascensions but tonight she calls for something that entirely blows my mind.

'Where is Peter?' she asks.

This name, not a pet or a person I know of, is troubling. I don't want to keep repeating myself about dementia, but it does play on one's mind whenever something seemingly untoward arises, which is every ten minutes or so. She trundles off (I am carrying all her stuff at this point and so, for once, am less able). She comes back toting an old doll's head from who knows where.

Peter, it turns out, was her childhood toy, beloved since the late 1920s, and his severed noggin is still deployed in times of trouble for support and comfort. I've been back here thirteen months and spent eighteen years living with her, but I have never seen or heard of Peter before. Yet here he is, dark-eyed and ghostly pale. My mother holds him out, as though playing Hamlet.

'I am like him,' she announces.

She tilts Peter's porcelain head and his eyelids fall.

'I lie back, I close my eyes.'

Then she climbs the stairs, Peter's head under her arm like a cartoon phantom. I am touched. Upset, I suppose. Afraid to lose her. I am a child again. When I see my folks as kids, and sometimes it shines through so clearly, I wonder what it says about who we are underneath all this accumulated and invisible time and expectation. Stretched and desiccated babies. Baffled by a race we never meant to run.

This Is Ourselves

I use the old tricks of luring Dad back to better mobility through tea and whisky. If he asks for a brew I suggest we make it together. Then he tries it alone. When the six o'clock Scotch call comes this is conditional on his independence. And so he rises, more each day, raising the bottle of malt like a dumbbell. Though he continues to hide from the physio as artfully as the Apache in his daily Westerns . . . he is improving.

I see flashes of character returning. The human being, not just the old, embattled thing. He makes a great, well-timed joke.

'What's the plan today, then?' asks my mother one morning.

'I'll get out there and mow the lawn,' he answers.

He may well weigh less than the mower.

He is back on his tablet too. Smashing out food orders that have nothing to do with anyone else's diet or the one he should be following. We are back where we started, which is better than where we've been.

A sign of quite how far we've come but might yet stumble is that Mum is talking about driving. It's been five months, and part of me had hoped she just wouldn't fancy it. When the snow melts she is soon fondling the car keys and staring hungrily up the road like Senna, or the *Great Escape* version of Steve McQueen.

As a non-driver I recuse myself from the arguments around this, which would be intense, if my brother actually engaged in them. Action over discourse is more his scene, for better or worse.

The rattle of car keys is overrun by the thud of hooves that heralds the arrival of my sister's chariot of catastrophe. She runs a filibuster, arguing that Mum should throw in the towel before something happens. I suggest Mum take an assessment course. Then one day my brother simply gets in the car with her and they ride around the block and neighbourhood until he declares her match fit.

It is less her well-being that I fear for than that of others. That she might hurt someone seems an unbearable outcome. Mentally I compose a note to the parents of a squashed child saying, 'Sorry, but I'm the youngest so it's not my fault. Yours, a forty-seven-year-old man.'

Mum's first forays are tentative. I accompany her. It feels much like driving with her last year. No better or worse. She has a fascination with aircraft vapour trails that can cause her to take her eyes off the road. Certain plants and flowers will claim her attention.

'Oh, magnolia!' she will cry, as she veers towards the wrong lane.

Last year she took both hands off the wheel for emphasis while driving down a dual carriageway, turned to me and announced –

This Is Ourselves

'I love this car!'

'PUT YOUR HANDS ON THE WHEEL AND LOOK AT THE ROAD!'

She is almost always signalling, and she can't park. Apart from all that, it's OK. Besides, there is nothing like driving slowly to show you how frenzied everyone else is.

With Dad so much better and Mum at the wheel I accept another two weeks of teaching work and prepare to flee our rickety scene.

31 March 2018

On the day of my departure, having got the place up and running and admitted the district nurse, I take a belated shower. These delayed purifications have attained a sacred quality. If I am in the bathroom then the tough part of the day is usually behind us. Even if there is more to follow, these moments at least are my own. I have trained myself to set concern aside here and just marvel at the light on the water as it runs down the stall. This is another bright, south-facing room. I have music on. I look in the mirror and tell myself I am still in the game, pulling faces and tensing biceps like I'm seventeen. The teenage energy is compounded this morning since I am in a small way leaving home again, albeit only for a fortnight. But it is something, another step up the mountain towards somewhere else to be. At least I know and accept I'll be coming back this time. The illusion of permanence – in decisions, in anything, like the shower, drains away.

I am making the best of its low-pressure jets when Mum

bursts in – not unprecedented but usually held at bay with an amplified announcement that:

'I AM IN THE SHOWER!'

Not today. Mum lurches further into the room, repeating –

'Emergency! Emergency!' like a vehicle reversing.

Clearly this is serious. I throw on some clothes.

The district nurse explains that she has removed Dad's old catheter, but cannot get the new one in. There is an art to this. We take it for granted, but it doesn't just happen. No one else on her team is available, so we'll have to go to A & E. Dad isn't keen, but his kidneys will pack up otherwise, or something drastic and renal along those lines.

The nurse tells us to tell the reception at casualty that he is 'in retention'. I call a cab and we rattle down familiar roads to hospital. Despite his circumstances, we must still wait our turn among the injured builders, luckless kids and the who-knows-what-is-up-with-them-but-you-wouldn't-want-it crowd.

For all his intransigence, Dad is stoic when it comes to it. It is odd, I admire him in hospital but resent him at home. Also we talk more here, as though in the presence of a higher power that enables this. The pressure is off us, some-what. Sooner or later, someone will turn up and tell us what to do.

The higher power keeps us waiting for about an hour, then I wheel him through the action-packed and tech-heavy halls of the ICU into a cubicle where a Spanish nurse checks details and asks questions. The man takes a catheter and slides it precisely into Dad in one perfect, painless move.

'You should play darts,' I tell him.

This Is Ourselves

He doesn't smile, but he doesn't have to. What you need here is expertise. My search for bonhomie is my own problem.

In under two hours we are back home with the kettle on. When the healthcare system works it's beautiful. Exquisite. You can't believe it's there. Each encounter with it soothes him, I think. The experience beats the headlines every time.

The sense that our problems are soluble pervades the house, and we sit together in the living room and laugh about the life we lead. That it came to this. They thank me:

'It's very helpful.'

And somehow nothing else matters, the circumstances, the sickness and the fights and the shit . . . the bare blessing of having them both alive is all there is. All one could feel or wish for.

These fleeting benedictions after the battle are beyond words. This is not about quality of life, perhaps, but life itself. In its way this has been a mad second childhood, one you can better recall. Closer than the pale Polaroid memories in the albums upstairs. Far from the past yet somehow the same. We keep to our separate corners of the living room like the tired fighters we are. An old recurring constellation. If more of us could stand this might become a group hug.

'Come back and see us soon,' says Dad.

As if I had popped in for a visit, instead of living and hiding there for over a year. I think perhaps he misunderstands all this. But maybe he is setting me free. I kiss them both goodbye and call a cab. How I love them when I'm leaving. I wonder if this is nautical blood. A sailor's affliction. Did he use to feel the same? All the right feelings at all the wrong times.

The Son Also Rises

Spring yields subtle changes. I feel guilty when I am not with my parents. Until today. I phone while they are eating. Mum is back to cooking, both are enjoying proper food. What I am hoping for perhaps is another declaration of thanks: 'We're fine and it's all down to you.'

Instead, Mum, whom I had seen for so long as dependent and a thing to be defended, tells me to call back when they're done with dinner. Startling enough, but then she doesn't quite hang up the phone and I can hear them complain about me phoning.

'What's he thinking?'

'He knows this is a busy time.'

'We're trying to eat,' says my dad, as though he was emerging from Ramadan instead of the living room.

I keep listening, somewhat stunned. Offended, even. And then the real story hits me as I hear them grumble, clank and chew.

They have a life of their own, quite apart from me, 'us', and the problems that have become so ingrained in my perception that I see projections of woe instead of people. People who just want to eat without answering the phone. My head is turned around. This is no grievance. This is great news.

20 April 2018

I am borrowing my friend in Africa's flat again, an arrangement that causes me to meet a Gambian friend of his, Hassoum. We are in a hotel bar when Hassoum asks me what I do. I say I mainly look after my folks. The standard British response to this, which I have become accustomed to, is somewhere on the empathy/pity spectrum.

Hassoum, conversely, looks at me as if I have just become a father (not metaphorically inaccurate, perhaps), does a kind of fist-pump gesture and announces –

'This is a great thing to do!'

I marvel at the cultural contrast. Then he tells me he has ten children, so he is belt and braces with this stuff, at least when he has his trousers on. He may have a better attitude, but he is also working the odds. One of them is bound to look after you.

26 April 2018

News from home. Dad has shingles. It's on his back and in his eye. This is the condition that laid Mum up for months, pain lingering in her nerves. I think it might do for him, or at least lay him very low indeed. I concede that the window of freedom might be falling again.

I am as geared up to return as Dad is to get sick (this, as ever, is the key difference between them; Mum had further to fall), when Dad does something un-Dadlike, and recovers in days. By the time I get back his skin looks furious but the man inside is on the mend. As ever, none of this is predictable. If this were a casino game you would walk from the table, bankrupt and amazed. Yet on we play.

3 May 2018

A week later you would never know it happened. The sun is out and we are back into some kind of functionality. I will continue to come and go, a week here and then a week away. This seems an amenable balance. None of us has to cut the cord completely and face who we are alone. Like a house of cards that seems to settle into its own structure, life appears to stabilize.

17 May 2018

Early signs of summer set off something in the Old Man's mind. He has ordered a white suit online. He has no memory of this when it arrives, but I salute the intention even as my sister returns it. Wherever he thought he might get to in these garments, it is a dream he wasn't having months ago.

Mum keeps to her minimal driving regimen. She doesn't taxi her mates about as much as she once did, but she does enough to stay free in her own perception. As with Dad and the unworn clothes, the idea is more important than what we might tyrannically assert as one another's reality – the fuels and labour that underwrite these cheap linen and petroleum dreams notwithstanding.

Back on the Drain Gang

5 June 2018

It's hot now. Almost enough to turn the heating off. Heady days. I am mindful of the house itself, which seems to creak and stretch as it too tries to shrug off winter. Like the bodies of its tenants, the homestead has had enough.

This is especially true of the drains, which sometimes pack up altogether and flood back into the house through the toilet, the consequences of which are exactly as you would imagine. Despite being a fastidious neurotic in some regards, the last fifteen months mean that my prior reservations about dealing with sewage have evaporated.

Deciding what to repair in an elderly household is a daily dilemma. I can't even screw in a light bulb without wondering if it will last longer than those it illuminates. The Old Man has his *Do Not Resuscitate* notice ready for when he next malfunctions. Most things I try to revive rather than replace. Piecemeal drain repairs are now my speciality.

If I don't prise up the cover and drop down with the garden hose every twelve weeks or so, the drain will buckle. I have a reminder on my phone about this. Even so, I miss my slot and then, this shimmering June afternoon, it happens again.

My parents call me to the living room.

'It's the toilet.'

I know what this means, but somehow, like a player trapped in some endless production, I step through the dialogue anyway.

'What's up with it?'

'It's overflowing.'

'What's been going on?'

They fend me off together over this stuff; the denial is choral.

'Nothing.'

'Nothing.'

'We don't know.'

Soon I have access to hard evidence – the impacted knot of excrement, wipes and paper that one must blindly chisel free from the drain like some cursed sculptor. And yet, when I resume the inquisition as to whose reckless self-purification is to blame, I am reminded of another shocking truth of our household – everyone lies. The three of us together are over two hundred years old, yet we fib about the toilet.

The web of deception was first clear to me when my parents' counter-intelligence operation about which of them eats short-bread collapsed last summer. Diabetes isn't even in the Premiership of the Old Man's ailments, but it's there, and along with certain other comorbidities isn't helped by the substitution of biscuits for 'proper' food. Plus, if I clean up your shit, I should get a say in what you eat, perhaps.

The persistence of shortbread despite my never buying it

meant of course that someone was. Though they are obsessed with the stuff, neither can quite remember its name. So they call it 'the Scottish biscuit', like superstitious actors afraid to speak the title of their play.

Each blames the other for the purchase and accuses the other of eating it. Then one day I was at the shop with Mum and she stuck some in the trolley. I asked who it was for, pointed out that Dad was in hospital and she just shrugged and tottered off towards the eggs. I knew then the calamitous truth. They were both eating it. And they were both lying. Denial and desire entwined, with me, like some doomed detective in this biscuit noir, never quite grasping the wider game.

So it goes with the drains.

'Not me,' says one.

'I would never,' insists the other.

'The carers throw stuff down there,' they assert together.

The many mad battles that might make up the day are yours to pick, and sometimes my internal CPS lets us all off the hook by assessing that there is nothing to be gained from prosecution, and we can let the whole thing drop.

But the drains are the drains. It's £300 to get it done if I'm not there. And then there is the 'shame' (Mum's words, not mine) of the Dyno-Rod van parked outside.

'A bright orange thing!' She shudders as she recalls it.

I do not share her misgivings, but I know they are deeply enough felt that she cannot be the problem. I know whose behind is behind it. Equally, I am so relieved when the culprit makes it to the toilet, let alone on their own, that these missions to the midden are a small price to pay.

Back on the Drain Gang

Plus, I get to feel hands-on and useful. Down here I am a fixer, not a thinker. And when one does a thing entirely, one is just the doing of the thing. A strange freedom lurks in such neglected spaces. Even in the often-blocked drain.

Mum looks on as I hose off my boots, having beaten the obstruction.

'You had a lot of badges in the Scouts,' she muses.

Two, actually. Reading and lighting fires. Both matters I still hold dear.

'Is there a badge for this?'

'There should be.'

Brighter Later

The sun keeps coming. The house and garden transformed from winter now. As she inspects her flowers Mum is in reflective mood.

'Six months on I can look back on it, being so unwell,' she says.

She talks of Christmas, which we took as a success, getting them out of the house and all the rest of it. She says she felt so awful that she spent the journey to my brother's praying that the traffic lights didn't change, that it would all be over quicker and so home again. I sensed nothing of this at the time, adrift in my own concerns.

'I feel I should warn people,' says Mum, about old age.

'Just live on and well as an example,' I say, a little too quickly. Maybe I am speaking less for her here than for myself.

27 June 2018

A deeper past is invoked by the World Cup. My parents are old enough to feel pleasure whenever Germans fail, and the football duly delivers. An echo of even older battles arises when, since we are now lurching up the hierarchy of needs, out of the survival zone and into the cosmetic, a man comes to clean the patio.

'He has a chemical from America,' says Mum, repeatedly. 'A chemical from America.'

It seems to me just to be chlorine, and a vapour cloud rises across the garden and glides into the house. My folks appear immune to this, but I can hardly inhale, and my eyes are streaming. I run outside, to die on the lawn perhaps, like something witnessed by a poet from the First World War.

I am still melodramatically fighting for breath when my mother comes out, ignores me and admires the now bleached patio.

'I can't believe it,' she says.

The mould on the stone has been a consistent source of woe for her, even in much harder times. Strange what the mind returns to. Never mind your choking son.

'How long will this last?' she asks the American chemical (chlorine) man.

'Four years,' he says.

'Four years,' she says to Dad excitedly. 'We're in the clear!'

She doesn't think they'll live that long. I cough up more poison from my lungs. All bets are off, I think.

3 July 2018

Having survived patio Passchendaele, I have a more positive Germanic interaction when a friend lures me into town. A new art gallery has risen from the ruins of an old department store and its images do our city and my spirits proud. I have always loved art and understand people's anxieties over public spending on it, but I can say this. These abstract patterns are so far aside from the outer reality of my life that something deeper in me rises to meet them. It is healing.

We visit the city's older gallery. The same pictures have hung here all my life and so offer something on each return. Another means to know oneself. I come home buoyant at the power of art on the ailing mind. I see my folks' clutter anew. There must be some voodoo power they get from all this, the gallery of their lives.

5 July 2018

Dad's eighty-eighth birthday is coming. Having bought almost everything that he has ever seen advertised he can be tough to find presents for, but I am thinking of getting him something to do with his old hometown. I'm on the Internet when I discover he grew up next to what was then Europe's highest industrial chimney, known as 'the Audley Destructor'. It looks astonishing, unreal in pictures, dwarfing cars and people. Higher than the Statue of Liberty.

Over three hundred feet tall.

I ask him what it was like, imagining this would be an indelible thing, as powerful in his recollection as it is exciting to me in discovery.

'Yeah,' he says. 'It was just sort of there.'

It cuts both ways, the world of value. My Dad has two

things he repeatedly returns to, and all I do is let the repetition annoy me. One is a picture above the mantelpiece, a rural scene of the Yorkshire moors, purchased on a driving holiday in the mid eighties. I was spoiled by foreign travel and alive with hormones at the time. Driving through Yorkshire wasn't my idea of fun.

'You know that picture?' he starts.

Yup, I know the picture. And then he will either praise the picture, or the holiday, or the living room, itself a cluttered pantheon of days gone by. And then all this happens again. The sulking teen, in some measure, remains.

'YES, I KNOW THE F*CKING PICTURE!' I think. But it emerges as a mutter.

Sorry, please forgive me. Press restart.

We have a similar ritual with a place mat depicting a Lancashire hotel where we would gather with extended family years ago. The house has many photos of this scene; folk, fashions and cigarettes all long gone.

He holds the place mat up after dinner and says –

'You won't remember this place . . .'

But I do and always did, and now it seems important to him to remind me once again. This happens a lot.

'You know we went through this last week?' I used to ask.

He seems admonished, but it is a tough thing to reckon, what to accept and what to fight for. You don't want them to slide too easily to the place where they don't know what's what any more. That, in part, might be what I am defending when my patience goes. On better days I tell him the name of the hotel.

'Oh,' he says, almost unconcerned, 'is that what it was called?'

Feelings beat details these days. I have long had that the wrong way around.

Ill Communication

Drunk on the idea things might not be so bad after all, my siblings and I hatch a plan. My sister turns sixty in mid July and is gathering her friends in Spain. If we all go, this will be the first time we have left our parents without one of us on hand for nearly two years. It should work. Dad has the carers, Mum is driving well, and is well in part because she is driving. They have their alert-call necklaces. The neighbours are vigilant. My sister lends me money and I book a flight. I need a holiday. Arguably from my family, eighty per cent of whom will be alongside me, but any resort in a storm . . .

A challenge to all this arises almost instantaneously when my parents' landline fails. Eschewed by some households, this old-fashioned system remains the spine of theirs. The alert-call system runs through the landline, as does the broadband which has vanished into the bargain. They both have basic mobiles but neither like nor especially understand them. The signal at the house is poor, too. We can't leave them here with nothing.

Neither, you might think, could the phone company, but no. Their clients' vulnerability is no obstacle to the baroque opera of disinformation, institutionalized indifference and psy-ops-level bullshit that ensues as we attempt to get reconnected.

Our first point of contact is an overseas call centre. Nothing against those per se, but in this instance they are evidently predisposed by the same corporate connivance and cost-cutting that engenders their existence to tell us lies.

'The whole street is down,' one operator tells me, assuring me this large-scale crisis is being considered at the highest level.

I go next door; the neighbour's phones are fine. I call back; different operator, ten minutes of explanations to establish the same untruth (all this from my mobile, with poor reception).

'The whole area is affected!' says the operator, sounding alarmed now at the scale of the outage.

'It's not,' I say. 'I've been next door.'

'You are mistaken.'

'I'm not mistaken.' With that, they hang up.

My anger at this could defrost a turkey.

I quash this inner Chernobyl with a few deep breaths and a futile kick of the kitchen table. Like the real Chernobyl, these early countermeasures can but mask a deeper problem. The idea that this kind of barefaced arseholery is now our lot in life and more so at the end of it . . . the heat of that will not quite die away. The heat of that might be why I am writing. Why I pick up the phone again.

Having dismantled Lie A, I am now presented with Lie B.

'There are problems at the dig.'

My parents' neighbourhood is uncommonly silent in the July heat and if you hit a soft-boiled egg with a hard spoon round here, I, even through tinnitus, would be aware of it. No one is digging.

'Where is the dig?' I ask.

They don't know.

'I have a bicycle and lots of time. Tell me where the dig is, and I'll take them a flask of tea.'

'The whole area is down.'

'No, it isn't.'

They put me on hold. Then the signal dies.

This goes on and on. No explanation of my parents' vulnerability makes any difference. None of the reasons I am offered makes sense.

'Can you send us an email?' says someone at the call centre.

'No,' I repeat. 'There is no broadband, nothing.'

'Oh,' they say, as though this were a surprise.

9 July 2018

Each futile call takes around fifteen minutes, if they don't hang up on me or I don't lose the signal. I have made five to ten of these a day for two days. Today I complain on social media, another world completely inaccessible to my parents. I go a bit over the top, in public, but the response is instantaneous.

Someone phones me from the UK. They are very sorry. Because my parents have not applied, by post and via their GP, for vulnerable status, they cannot be treated as such.

'So this is how you treat everyone else?'

That a simple request should expose one to the full force of contemporary corporate aggravation is just one of the everyday outrages of elderly life. Again, I must reflect and record that without someone as time-rich and pathologically intransigent as me on their side, they, and others like them, would be done for. I make a big speech about this to Mum and Dad as they sit in the living room, since *a)* it is about them, and *b)* who else would listen?

'What's he talking about now?' says Mum to Dad when I've finished.

He shrugs. I go back to my room.

14 July 2018

After eight days of isolation and chicanery which are now threatening to jeopardize the holiday, an engineer comes. In a world of call centres and systemic indifference, a visit from a human is like water in the desert, and the heat makes this even more so. He spray-paints symbols on the shimmering drive. Mum looks on, impressed.

'These are men,' she pronounces. 'The others who came were boys.'

'What others?'

'Oh, some people came the other day while you were out, I didn't think to tell you.'

That I have been screaming of injustice without the facts is galling, to say the least. But it doesn't matter. The real man comes back with other real men. They fix it in an hour.

Ill Communication

15 July 2018

The phone company call me back, asking me if I am satisfied. I just want to know that my complaint is registered, that this might happen less, if it ever has to happen again.

'It's registered, absolutely.'

'Then read it back to me.'

'We can't do that without a Freedom of Information request.'

I give up and go to Spain.

Holiday, Celebrate

18 July 2018

Three days into our trip my brother beckons me across the villa in the manner of someone wanting to share drugs without alerting the rest of the party. Instead he has news from home.

Dad has fallen and broken his femur. He is back in hospital. Mum called an ambulance and John has stepped into the breach and is keeping things together. All things considered, this is a contained crisis. No need to fly home. No sense in telling our sister, who celebrates her birthday unencumbered by the news. Her 'hip, dementia, death' refrain rattles through my mind as the week goes on. Things were going so well.

I might be on a beach, but beyond the blue horizon I am more than ever conscious of how fate carefully folds our plans and drop-kicks them into the bin. To clear my head I rent an expensive mountain bike. An astonishing machine, the best I have ever ridden.

'Where are you planning to go?' asks the lender.

'Away from my family,' I say.

How we laugh.

Holiday, Celebrate

21 July 2018

This morning I am due to return the bike. I leave it locked outside for thirty seconds while I grab my wallet. When I look down from the balcony, it's gone. When I get down to the street it is still missing. As is my sense of reality. I am gutted, more so than by Dad's fall and what this might mean for our conjoined futures. Or maybe the fear of that is playing out in this.

The man in the bike shop confirms that he hasn't stolen it as a prank, which was my last hope. We're not laughing any more. I find myself telling God directly that I get the message. Then the man in the shop tells me I am not insured. I don't have time to go to the police because I need to get to the airport. When I get there, we are moved on and off the same plane repeatedly like an experiment in crowd psychosis.

I watch the rest of my extended family leave unhindered through the glass walls of the gate where I'm detained. Until my flight is eventually cancelled. The delay is several hours, which pass like days. I come to think of Alicante airport as home.

23 July 2018

At actual home, the familiar juxtaposition of peace and regret reigns as it always does when the Old Man is in hospital. The carers are on indefinite hold and Mum seems pleased with the way she has handled the emergency, as well she should be. For Dad's part, he too is remarkably upbeat. They operated immediately and filled his thigh and femur with metal, 'gamma nailing' to avoid a wholesale hip replacement. They say he will walk again, but he was barely managing to begin with. We shall see.

As ever, the outcome of this latest twist (to think of them as setbacks is to imply a forward motion which, as Spain has taught me, again, is the way of fools) will affect our world at large. If he can't walk, then what? He also has a case of hospital-acquired pneumonia. It says something about us and our situation that this feels like no big deal.

The fact I'm back again is fine with me. To see my attempts to rejoin society unravel so entirely at the hands of a bicycle thief is all the excuse I need to throw in the beach towel and pick up the wipes. Besides, it's sunny. I love the summer here. I would come home at this time of year and sit in the garden anyway. The hell with progress and ambition and socially sanctioned self-regard. If the world needs me, I'll be on the patio.

Meantime, familiar patterns emerge. The physios announce themselves and I expect once again to hold their version of my father's fitness against what might actually work at home and then fight to reconcile these disparate visions. That is weeks away. For now, he can't even stand.

Carry on Screaming

24 July 2018

The hospital is hot, filled with fans to which we add as many as his corner can sustain. His neighbours are fractured and fractious. A young man who's been in a scooter accident yells. Says he is in constant pain. The others on the ward, all elderly, have had their sympathy devoured by this noise, and now view him with collective generational disdain. Even his mother looks annoyed with him. Who are we, to judge each other's screaming? Nevertheless, it is great when he shuts up. Not for the first time, I reflect on how kind thoughts fashioned at a distance are often withered by proximity to the problem.

25 July 2018

So it goes at the homestead. Mum and I sip drinks on the patio in the long evenings, reflecting on the garden, time and old age. Everything is easier close to nature. Freudian paradise regained. Mum gains some independence, mastering the TV remote control for the first time. We meet for meals but otherwise I come and go as I please, though mostly to the hospital.

Dad has shrugged off the pneumonia and says scooter boy's screaming is driving him crazy. This he says out loud since it is the consensus of the ward. Then he waves me closer for an off-the-record aside.

'They're not giving me my temazepam,' he says. 'Bring some from the house.'

I check with the ward sister who consults a list and says he is absolutely getting the drugs.

'I don't want to give you drugs the doctors don't know about,' I tell him.

The doses are specific. He's on a huge, and one must presume carefully counterbalanced, cocktail as it is.

'They're not giving me the right pills.'

'They say they are.'

He looks me in the eye, that rarest of things, and says –

'Trust your father.'

This feels like a moment from a movie neither of us are actually in, and certainly not together. I confess I don't trust him, in this regard especially. I give it up to the higher power, the hospital, on this one. Again, this is one of the upsides of having him here. You are free of the burden of having to figure out exactly what to do.

Not content with nailing a near-ninety-year-old back together, the NHS yields another miracle even as it seems to stumble and stagger itself. One of the physio team is also my sister's next-door neighbour. I can't say that this confers any special treatment, and indeed would hope not, but the cycle of having him thrust back on us prematurely in the usual high-stakes game of pass-the-pensioner is broken when we are informed that Dad qualifies for residential rehab at the smaller hospital across town.

As far as I can tell there are eight of these beds for men in a city of over 250,000 people. This feels like a lottery win. We have wished for this before, many times, and now it has been granted. He will have at least three weeks of dedicated care aimed at helping him to walk again. We can expect a man who can move by himself and we may make the most of the interim. Dad is pleased, but I can see that this is bittersweet for him. All he really wants is to come home.

4 August 2018

The new place is peaceful. No one on his ward calls out in pain or dementia. Dad has a TV and a window. Good as all this is, the improved circumstances have an unforeseen if entirely predictable outcome. After some disappointing early forays towards the toilet (as ever the porcelain grail of recovery), the physios here inform us that it is as if he'd prefer not to move at all.

'They're on to him,' says my sister, with the hollow certainty of one who has had an old, uncomfortable suspicion confirmed.

I imagine this is like working hard to get your child into further education and then discovering they spend most of their time in bed or on drugs or both. In that sense, touché, Old Fella. Turnabout is fair play.

15 August 2018

Dad seems miffed that this 'is not a hospital ward', as the staff remind him when he expects more comprehensive assistance. I visit expecting to find him sitting or walking, but he is mostly prone. Likewise, I come with the intention of having a useful or important conversation, but find these ideals equally flattened by the silences which transpire instead.

Not always. Sometimes he has wisdom to live by.

'When you're young,' he says to me, 'sex is the main thing . . .'

I can sense the qualifying clause approaching and hang expectantly on the punchline.

'When you're old . . .' Here it comes . . . 'it's all about opening your bowels.'

In the end you need a partner for both. Dad's mismatched accomplice is a no-nonsense male nurse who must be sixty himself, but radiates and manifests remarkable strength, physical and mental. He could, I suspect, carry Dad to the bathroom in the palm of his hand but absolutely will not do so. Instead they explore a prolonged antagonistic duet in which he patiently goads and encourages my father to do things for himself.

Dad hates it, wants me to complain about him, but I won't. As far as I'm concerned, the man is a hero, a drone for my deepest desires, and we are living vicariously through his indifferent determination. I'm not sure what the reverse of Nietzsche's 'will to power' is – will to bed? will to biscuits? – but my father's embodiment of this is steadily being overturned. Again we might call for music and cut to montage. Again there is progress.

Beyond Retro

I bring Mum in a cab and they sit together. I have no idea quite what passes between them at these times, they are like the last two believers of some ancient faith. Speakers of some lost, inaudible tongue. Their love, if it is that, does not submit to rational analysis. It is their business. So I leave them to it, I fetch teas. I walk about the hospital.

I was a patient here myself once, for months. In another life, it seems. Mum was too distressed, I think, to see me unwell to visit often. Dad came almost every day. My wife too. The pain of that long incarceration is just as vanished as the many pleasures since. Who are we, I wonder, if we can't hold on to what seemed once to be our notable days? We must be more than the details, and even the feelings.

A woman on the next ward is distressed with dementia, calling out for details long gone. And yet sometimes she seems serene in ways I can only wish for. Is this because she has remembered, or because she no longer cares?

This building is dense with memories. Mum worked here as a volunteer at one time. As a teenager I once crawled through the lobby on all fours to avoid being spotted by her while I was receiving treatment for venereal disease. It is also the central psychiatric hospital, so crawling about is largely overlooked.

18 August 2018

Another factor of Dad's absence is that Mum can take visits from friends who are otherwise deterred by the behavioural exclusion zone that ordinarily emanates from his occupied chair. One lady comes over and they chat in the garden for a long time. I am not trying to eavesdrop, but they are working at volume. The conversation eventually peters out, and after a prolonged exchange of filler – 'Hmm', 'Well', 'Yes', 'So', stops entirely.

'Well, I'd best go and visit him,' says Mum, eventually.

I've already been and my sister's going later, so there is no need. I run outside and announce this, thinking I am doing a good thing.

'You don't need to go in today, Mum.'

Mum shakes her head at me, frantically but discreetly. I worry she's having a seizure, then realize what is going on.

With nowhere else to be and no one to hurry them, she and her friend have talked themselves to a standstill, and Mum is making stuff up now to get her to leave. This must be a thing with old people. With time on your hands, you run out of excuses. Nothing, however boring, need actually come to an end. A hidden hell. Now I have blown the con. I feel awful. I phone the landline from my mobile and Mum answers.

'Hello?'

'It's me.'

'Who?'

'Your youngest child.'

'But you were just here.'

'I still am. I'm on the other phone.'

'Why?'

'So you can pretend this is something important.'

'What?'

'PRETEND THIS IS IMPORTANT.'

'Ahh.'

She gets it now, as will the neighbourhood. Her friend leaves. Job done.

Dog Day Afternoon

21 August 2018

The rehab unit are precise about how much Dad should be able to do. To make sure the house is in tune with their expectations about how far he can seat and raise himself, they come around and measure everything. They decide that his chair, literal and figurative seat of his power for the last two decades, is too dangerous for him now since it swivels if you lean on it.

John comes over with his tools and we manage to de-swivel the chair. There is no time to celebrate as his dog, the Jack Russell with an instinct for finding holes and a knack for getting stuck down them, escapes into and then out of the garden. We walk the neighbourhood, calling her name, but there is no response. We split up.

I climb over a fence into the garden of a neighbouring house I thought was empty, but instead there is a young woman sunbathing on the lawn. She has a dog of her own lounging beside her, which I trust defuses some of the potential weirdness of my tumbling in here calling another's name. She is helpful and understanding but hasn't seen any Jack Russells. I am chiefly dumbfounded that she actually exists, that this isn't a mirage. No one under forty lives round here any more. I feel as if I am in one of Tony Soprano's dreams.

The hallucinatory vibe abides as I work my way higher up the hill onto an abandoned building site and clamber atop a wall. I can see all around from here, and the sunbathing neighbour has vanished. I call the dog's name and listen. No sound or sign of her, but there is something sublime in the silence, in the view of the neighbourhood, a subtle, wondrous instant. Have our problems flown, like that determined bird that fought its own reflection all winter long in the living room window? Or are they just on holiday?

This moment of apparent perfection is pierced by a familiar sound: my mum and sister arguing. The strange acoustics of the neighbourhood and indeed the volume at which one must speak to Mum to make a point carry their fractured discourse up the hill.

They are fighting about what kind of drip-dry shirt Dad should wear in hospital, which of the shirts in the house are drip-dry, and whether Mum should or should not do any ironing. This is a timeless classic of the genre and a fine example of how the family dynamic spins love into calamity just as readily as the reverse.

It makes zero difference what Dad wears, but it is nice to ask him. Then everyone falls out about it, and whatever you take him he will then say is wrong. It is a simple three-act play, and Act Two rings out across the suburbs for the hundredth time. In the interval there is a bustle in the hedgerow and the dog appears. I signal John and we surround her, get her back on the lead and inside, where the shirt, finally agreed on, hangs ready to be hospitalized.

I drop it off that evening. As ever, I go in wanting to save the world, to have the conversation that makes everything OK. As ever, this does not occur. I consider the famous cliché about the definition of insanity being expecting different outcomes from the same, repeated thing. I show him the shirt.

'That's not the one I meant,' says Dad.

He's in bed, but assures me he has been up and walking, somewhere between Chris Bonington and the risen Christ, if only I had been here half an hour ago to see it. I tell him we have fixed his chair so he can keep it. Praise me, I think.

'Can I have a biscuit?'

I trudge to the canteen to fulfil this familiar order where I notice a copy of a TV listings magazine with a starburst cover line: 'I've killed my Dad!' I take a shot of that on my phone, send it to my siblings with the qualifier: 'over some biscuits'. Cathartic emoji laughs ensue.

Back at the bedside I hand over the calories. The Old Man remembers he has news.

'I have tinnitus,' he announces.

'No, I have tinnitus,' I assert, defensively. I don't want him to have tinnitus. Tinnitus is mine.

'I can hear this noise,' he says.

'It's probably the TV,' I tell him.

A flat screen hangs over the bed like a physician. I can hear it humming from here. Plus he listens on headphones, which won't help. I outline these factors, but he is having none of it. He has tinnitus, he has told the doctors and now they are making fresh appointments for him.

I am so profoundly fucked off by this point that I am aware

that the idiot, the one expecting anything different ever, is always me. Like some undefeated end-of-level boss in a video game, he has exposed my weakness again. I must practise more. Go back to the beginning. I make a voice note in my phone to talk to my therapist about all this, get on my bike and go home. Again.

Walking Wounded

25 August 2018

Despite the everyday dysfunctions and the old hypochondriac Ninja moves, after twenty-one days of rehab Dad is fitter and more able than before his fall. It is remarkable what he can do now. He doesn't seem to see it, or feel it, but from the outside it is wondrous. He walks further and straighter and stronger, albeit on a frame again. It's like the ascent of man.

This would not and could not have happened at home. If he had come here straight from hospital he would likely have sunk more profoundly into his chair. As it is, this is a man that can be cared for and cooperate, should he choose to. In another blessed turn of events I get some teaching work over the day he is due to be discharged. Not enough to propel me into some bright new future, but it will get me back to London and pay for the stolen bike. More to the point, they can manage without me, I believe. The carers will pick up as before since he is no worse off than when he was admitted. As we understand now but must remind ourselves each time, the transitions are the hard part. Find the plateaus and peace can be known.

'There is no end to it,' says Mum this morning in a flicker of despondency as I am leaving.

'Well,' I say. 'There is.'

28 August 2018

My brother helps Dad out of hospital. My sister emails me after a couple of days.

'He is calling out for Eccles cakes.'

Months of worry, unquantifiable expertise, patience and state expense condensed into the call for confectionery. Business as usual. The sugar siren is home.

5 September 2018

A week later I am back in the saddle, keeping an eye on things, when the tinnitus appointment rolls around. They want to syringe his ears, and this can't happen at home so he must make it down to the GP, which ought not to be a problem. But problems where there ought not to be is how things tend to go.

Despite his record levels of fitness and the fact that I have a sheet, a manifest of his mobility from the hospital, stating exactly what he can and cannot do, when the cab comes, he refuses to move. Says he won't go, doesn't feel up to it. My brother is here.

'Look, there are two of us to help you. All you have to do is get to the door. You can totally do this.'

'No. No,' he says, and looks away.

Somewhere between the fact that he is demonstrably and

officially capable of making this journey and that I don't believe he is even suffering from the ailment he claims to be, I almost lose it. I say, in a calm voice whose construction is effort enough to make me want to scream –

'You know where this goes. If you won't work with us, when all we try and do is help you, someone else will look after you, and it won't be someone with your DNA and it won't be in this house.'

He just shrugs. My brother looks at me, asking, I think, for no escalation. I move to another room. No flashes of divine light on the carpet this time.

I apologize to the cab driver, who tells me his Dad is the same. We laugh and in that instant the wrath dissolves again. And again I ask myself what are these feelings that seem so compelling, but don't last? There is nothing specific to the anger that I feel in those moments, it is the wrath of all time. Molecular frustration. You could do anything with it, tear down buildings and breathe fire. I want out, for all our sakes. There must be a better way.

I go to pay the driver, but he says it's fine and drives away.

I open the post. There is a leaflet about diabetes. 'Being sedentary,' it warns, 'can lead to premature mortality.' How do you sell that to someone who's eighty-eight? My father goes back to bed, twice the distance of getting to the front door. He never mentions tinnitus again.

So he is medically better, but psychologically unchanged. And then it hits me, whether prompted by therapy or by the simultaneous aggregation of my own frustrations, that I might be barking up the wrong tree here.

Walking Wounded

I find a picture upstairs of Dad watching me carefully as a child, perhaps even fearfully, as I play near water. I need to go downstairs and see that man again, not the presenting illusion. I have a postcard too from him to me when I was very young. He's signed it 'Daddy', that familiar name I once asserted that we never used. Who am I fooling here and what for? I find something else amongst my souvenirs. A ticket stub from 1992, the last time we went to the movies together: *Unforgiven*.

PART FOUR

How Can Man Die Better?

10 *September 2018*

Little by little, we get over ourselves. I calm down. Dad admits to and embraces his recovery. One evening some veg falls from his plate and rolls towards Mum. He points it out with his fork and says –

'Bring me that truant pea.'

She flicks it towards him, and he forks it playfully into his mouth. On one level this isn't much, this comic duet. But in context it is a salutation, proof of life. Like seeing a band get back together that should never have broken up.

15 *September 2018*

Mum's ninetieth is approaching. The archives are out in preparation. She studies old photographs, which sets her in reflective mood.

'I didn't realize I was so nice-looking.'

My sister sends me a picture of Dad leading a conga line on a ship in the fifties. I have never seen him dance, but it's nice to know it happened.

21 September 2018

Dad's body isn't keen on reunions. It wants to split up. I am teaching again when my sister phones to tell me he is back in hospital, less than a month since he came out. Some grim trifecta of gout, diabetes, and poor circulation has struck. His whole heel is suddenly an open wound.

It has become so bad so quickly – a grade four pressure sore – that the hospital is obliged to launch a safeguarding case against us and the carers in case there is neglect. The summer's work is undone. Spiritually, physically, totally. It is debatable whether he will keep the foot or ever walk again. This would be big news, but I have reached a point where I have managed my expectations almost out of existence. Almost.

22 September 2018

By the time I get to the hospital I just feel tired and sad and worried to be back here again. For him and me and all points in between.

As ever, whatever feelings one brings are quickly taken aside and mugged by the facts. Far from the prone spectre I expect, Dad is in motion. Wheeled past me on a hospital bed. Cheerful and forthcoming. Possibly on drugs.

'Crackles on my chest!' he calls out. 'Amy will fill you in.'

A nurse nods obligingly. He reaches out and hands me his mobile phone.

'Get some credit on that.'

He looks up at one of the porters.

'Pedro!'

The porter smiles.

'Pedro, this is my son.'

I come here thinking it's game over, and he's on first-name terms with everyone. He seems to be controlling the place, rather than it shaping him. It is reminiscent of the rare times I visited him at work. What does this mean? I take my book to the chapel and try to remember that this is not something that has to be 'figured out'. Take a fixed position and the world will brain you. Stay open, and you might get to try again.

Undertow

The exuberance doesn't last. Next time I see him he could be dead. Eyes closed; mouth open. I've seen deeper-breathing plants. I recall the death of my mother-in-law. One astonishing rally and then it was over. A leaflet in her hospice explained that this is often the way. It was close to Halloween. Families dressed as ghosts and devils to attend the dying. Quite a night.

24 September 2018

Dad has pneumonia again, on top of everything else. His mind seems weaker too. His memory appears to worsen, as if the walls and curtains here were stopping him from seeing or recalling any wider world. He barely talks. The doctors frown and confer, confounded by his spread of ailments. No one knows quite what to do.

Undertow

25 September 2018

G-Wing. Geriatric. We have been here before. Last year he was in, I think, this very bed one boiling afternoon when a heavily made-up harpist wheeled her instrument onto the ward for a therapeutic recital. I am not sure I had ever seen a harp before; they are enormous things. It seemed an odd choice, given its association with the afterlife and the proximity of the audience to it, many of them unconscious as she played.

Beautiful as it sounded, to awaken to this Celtic figure in Kabuki make-up would have been startling. Possibly fatal. The picture grew stranger still when the League of Friends arrived and poured tea into china cups and saucers that rattled in the old men's hands. They passed out trays of lurid cakes. It was profound yet psychedelic.

No sign of the harp this time, but there are other visions in the room. A man with dementia makes long, confessional accusations, and questions no one you can see.

'Have I changed?' he wonders. 'Did you love me? Jim was a brilliant man! Brilliant engineer. Made loads of money for Malcolm. Is that him there? He was good-looking. Tall. Liked blokes but loved women. My best friend. Elaine was cruel. She ruined two lives. I didn't love her. My ruination.'

As if his mind were setting fire to its secrets, just to see the smoke.

At home, we debate the future. We don't know its precise shape but we can take a guess at what is coming. It's not much of a game show any more. Safe to say upstairs is gone now, and showers with it. My brother is all for altering the house downstairs to make one there. My mother baulks at the upheaval. I don't know if you can rebuild the house every time you lose an inch of faculty. Add fresh white tiles for every word of woe. At this rate he would end up dying in the Taj Mahal.

This is ever the tendency of the men in our family: the silence, the grand gesture and the expense. Love, it strikes me now, belatedly, is a matter of degree more than display. The subtle over the spectacular. Presence over parades.

28 September 2018

In hospital the Old Man says he doesn't care if he never showers again. Neither do I, especially. His ennui is contagious. More so than any consequence of lapsed hygiene. The sense of 'why bother?' spreads. Besides, his morning ministrations with soap and flannel seem enough. Digestive dramas apart he is strangely scentless, like some giant hypo-allergenic pet, but with less Instagram potential.

At home the Ryder Cup highlights are on TV. Mum studies the screen, but her eyes are off the ball.

'No beer bellies on this lot,' she observes. 'They are all out playing golf.'

This might be a benign observation, but I have an inkling it is more deeply driven, up from the bunker of her being. It always irked her that Dad had no hobbies that involved unnecessary, voluntary movement. Our house backs onto the council golf course. I am sure she willed him on there in retirement, whether to gain a few hours of domestic dominion or in foresight of the ailments to come from such inertia, or both.

'Silly ball!' rails my mother at the screen.

Silly ball indeed.

Either way it isn't fair, this retro-fitting, while I sit on the sofa watching the big TV he paid for, with my mother, as she nudges towards a century. Judging a man born bereaved in the last one, who never knew his own mother. I asked him once in hospital as we held hands, thinking he was dying, if he thought of her at all, this unknown, essential woman. There was no hesitation. All he said was –

'All the time.'

Outlaws of Empathy

Trying to catch the right doctor in a vast hospital is, like fishing, a matter of patience, practice and, at times, survival. I am seasoned and time-rich in this regard and Mum, miraculously, compared to last year, is almost independent. So I pack a book, get on the bike early and wait for the doctors to make their rounds.

I am abetted by a ward sister I have come to know over the years. She doesn't so much go the extra mile as dwell there. She has sent us meds in a minicab that would have taken hours to wait for when Dad was ready for discharge, and many other game-changing small things besides. She is able, like many of the women I have met in her position, to wrangle and weave time from chaos, to pull rabbits from the hat of a system that says: 'There are no rabbits left, give up and go home.'

This is where you find them. Soft-hearted stoics are the thin front line here. After years of observation, frustration and inspiration (I have clocked up many NHS hours on my own account, thanks to a ruinous back, ringing ears, bloodshot eyes and a restless mind), I can say with certainty that this is not a fiscal economy in the strictest sense.

Outlaws of Empathy

This is a system run, enabled and sustained, beyond the numbers, by acts of care. The thoughtful sister, the persistent physio, the district nurse who asked me how I was; these are the moments and the outcomes that make the rest possible, bearable, and then worthwhile. It is the outlaws of empathy, breaking the rules and bending their schedules in the hospital and among the carers, who bring us quality of life.

All this rumbles through me as I watch the ward's business unfold. The sister lets me sit inside a room used for staff meetings and the sharing of bad news. I can watch the junction of two corridors and the doors of four wards from here, and so lurk like a highwayman, waiting for the doctors to show.

It is clear from this position what goes into keeping an ageing population around. Even the synchronized rotations of the patients – Dad included – to avoid bedsores is a fraught logistical ballet. No doubt things must change as the elderly tidal wave rises over our increasingly parlous and penniless youth, but handing these things over to the people who brought you understaffed and out-of-control prisons, food banks and franchised wars seems like an act of chronic societal self-harm.

This isn't just clear in hospital and at home, where we co-manage and part-fund what is, in effect, a frontier outpost of the NHS, but everywhere I go. Dave's partner is a midwife whose shift work escorting people into the world means that she sometimes falls asleep as soon as she gets through the door.

At the other end of life and on a different corner of the same long road, another close friend, Ron's mother, Helen, is in the latter stages of lung cancer. She was a doctor, a senior physician who joined the board of the hospital and then left in despair. She spends much of her remaining time lobbying for things to be done better, for old people in particular. The rest is consumed with elaborate palliative procedures she insists on performing herself at home and byzantine attempts to procure drugs which would elude anyone without such a fundamental and determined understanding of the system, and a healthy pension. You or I would be dead by now.

I sit with her sometimes and report on the outside world and she nods and testifies, hoarsely and profoundly, how things once valued and valuable have been steadily undone by egotists and profiteers who could no more take your pulse than they appear to have one.

I think of this while I wait on my father as he slumbers and groans in the hospital bed the politicians he admires would rather that he paid for.

I watch one system struggle as I struggle with my own.

Ordinarily my father's faith in medical professionals is so profound that he rallies at the sight of them. It is so tangible, this turnaround, that it can feel frustrating. I have a friend whose dog seems to love strangers far more than she who feeds him. I imagine that feels much the same.

With any medic's arrival comes a wave of unconditional credulity that would not arise were the same words to issue forth from simple mortals, or myself. To this end I have considered using an actor to dress as a doctor, come to the house and say exactly what I want my dad to hear.

★

When the doctors come this time things are different. Dad seems barely interested, elsewhere, and uncertain who has been to his bedside before or why he is in hospital. The doctors note this and I am taken aside for further questioning. I confess he is worse, mentally. They ask about the situation at home and I detect or perhaps project a heavier gravity in their silent response. The consultant lists the Old Man's comorbidities and it sounds like some valedictory résumé. It goes on and on. The heel, the foot and the leg are front runners for now. The big decisions lie with the vascular team, who will appear, but no one knows when.

I ask if there is much to do about the diabetes.

'Type two!' says Dad, reflexively. 'Diet.' Like he was a captured soldier accustomed to revealing this and nothing else.

The booze and biscuit tunnels beneath this response seem scarcely to support reason. Surely, even at this point, what we eat affects our health? The doctor gives me an old-fashioned look for one so young and says –

'At this stage, it is really a question of calories by any means necessary.'

As if on cue, the trolley of chocolate and crisps which comes a couple of times a day rolls onto the ward and the doctors step aside. The roaring subtext here, it seems to me, is let the dying man have a biscuit. As the snacks roll towards him, the Old Man's eyes grow wide.

'Your father has told us he doesn't want to live any more,' says the consultant as the man in question gulps down a digestive and shrugs.

No more subtext then, this is out in the open now. Death

has disrobed and walks boldly among us, like a mad tramp in a mall.

If Dad's mind and body seem to have reached an agreement in principle, how long will it take them to come to terms?

'He says he isn't depressed, and that he doesn't wish to come back to hospital,' the doctor continues.

Dad tears into a second biscuit. I can't even compute what this means. Actually, I can but I just don't want to. As much as he hates hospital, it is a break for those at home. If he has dug what's left of his heels in then what comes next will be a strange, immobile struggle. He can't walk and there is nowhere for us to run. Short of keeping him in a bouncy castle for the pressure sores, we are flat out of moves.

'Don't worry,' says the doctor. 'There's a lot we can do at home.'

All Lost in the Supermarket

2 October 2018

At the house we engage in the customary phoney war before this latest and perhaps last incarnation of Dad returns. Mum studies the paper, never afraid to pitch herself into the maelstrom of modern life. She shakes the broadsheet, which seems almost as big as she is, concluding, apropos of who knows what –

'I sometimes think I could run a pop-up bar.'

When the evening news comes on there has been a murder nearby. She looks at me.

'We're both here.'

I ask if she means that neither of us is dead, or neither of us did it.

'Either, really.'

3 October 2018

We must get to the shops, for life goes on. First Mum wants to change her trousers and fix her lipstick.

'You never know who you might meet.'

Indeed, and you never know which of these unnecessary trips upstairs will be the last, but we must allow it. The odds of her making it upstairs without stumbling seem diminished each day. Nothing to be done, except perhaps livestreaming it and taking bets.

Freedom to pursue that which does not seem sensible to others is a measure of one's quality of life. Up she goes, for the tenth time this morning, like some ailing but heroic device. As relentless as the Old Man seems resigned.

At the checkout I have to stop her from putting her card in the machine before everything has been scanned. This is something of a ritual.

'Not yet!'

'Now?' she asks, seconds later, like an excited child.

'Now!' I announce when the final box of Kleenex meets the last sustainable bag.

She is punching in the PIN when my mobile rings. It's one of the consultant's team. She is kind but frank, making sure I have grasped the situation, in so far is this is something that can be firmly held, which, it seems to me, down here at the shitty end of life's stick, is hardly at all.

'You should know,' she says, 'that a time will come when there is nothing more that we can do for your father.'

'I understand,' I say immediately, which is technically true, but as I thank her I am stabbed by a less familiar sensation.

A new sadness. Something ancient and heavy stirring, bursting like a bud in a time-lapsed film. A sudden unforetold shift in the internal tide. Funereal weather. With arms full of shopping it all comes at once.

All Lost in the Supermarket

I have noticed this before in life. We struggle to muster the appropriate emotions at the societally designated time. Kind thoughts loiter behind cruelty. Pain calls right after we have insisted we were fine. Here then is grief, hidden among the groceries. That sluggish yet stratospheric, formless feeling. I want to sink to my knees, but I am carrying a lot of eggs.

Here, at a supermarket till, not at any of the aborted bedside farewells or back-of-ambulance exchanges, the enormity of losing a parent hits home. Along with the crooked nature of human emotional progress. Things hurt when they hurt, not when they happen.

In the car park the woman who rounds up the trolleys and sings as she does so – something of a local celebrity – is strangely silent.

'She's normally singing, that one,' says Mum. 'Perhaps she's on some different tablets.'

At home I shake the sadness off, bury it in parts, like a body, and pack away the shopping, as one does. As billions do each day. I'm making dinner when Dad phones. He is going for an X-ray and is worried he doesn't have the right clothes.

'I don't think it matters what you wear for an X-ray, it's about your insides,' I say. 'As long as you aren't in lead-lined pants you should be fine.'

'I need clothes for the X-ray,' he repeats.

The idea won't shift any more than it will yield to logic. I go to the hospital. When I get there the X-ray has happened, and he has forgotten that we spoke.

'You know,' I say, 'just because you don't want to come to

hospital again, which I understand, that doesn't mean we can build a hospital at home.'

I forget what he says, and I expect he forgot that I said anything anyway, but I feel mildly better for saying it, which is sometimes enough. Maybe if we all switch off our minds we can make it through. Thinking won't fix this. That much stays true.

4 October 2018

Next morning I intercept one of the vascular team. She explains they would prefer not to operate again. Too risky. Instead Dad must keep his foot off the ground for all but an hour a day. His walking days are over, in effect. If the foot is low and doesn't heal then that might be the end of it, and perhaps the leg and him with it.

She hands me a giant plastic shoe, like a ski boot, which he will have to wear in bed. He won't be able to sit at a table, so he will need to be fed.

'How long might this go on for?'

'Several months,' she says. 'At least.'

There's nothing here that can be rehabbed. This will be the shape he comes back to us in, and he will be back soon. If he can't move except for getting up to the toilet, and that with assistance, then this is getting beyond what we can manage, even with carers to do the arising and bedtime business.

Given that he now forgets much more, including when and whether he has had his medication, it seems sensible, essential, to get more help. Unless I am prepared to make this my full-time occupation, which I know now, after eighteen months of dress rehearsal, method acting and several fleeting tastes of freedom, I would rather not.

I am conscious that in considering extending his professional care I am plotting my own escape, or at least underwriting its possibility. Although I know it chafes my parents' will to independence and even co-dependence, life is so much better with the carers there.

Capable, kind, dispassionate people coming in daily allows a level of therapeutic disengagement for us three children which adds an inestimable layer of sanity to one's day. I at least feel less like I live and sleep within millimetres of a spinning lathe, which is what I used to see when I closed my eyes.

The brittle matrix of possibilities that constitutes our lives, never more than a slip or a cough away from chaos, has been subtly cemented by outside help. I know people whose parents flat out refused assistance and lived in rising dirt and danger while their kids could only look in and look on. Dad's sliding health makes such outcomes impossible. There is a blessing in this somewhere, even if you need tweezers and a torch to find it.

So-Called Soul

Mum flinches when I suggest Dad will need four care visits a day. I explain if he is going to be at home, this is how it must be. It can't fall to her to monitor everything and to make him meals and then carry them through the house to him and help him to the bathroom. That would be the undoing of her, and then the whole thing would be in free fall.

'We have to accept this,' I say. 'Or I stay here and do everything, which even I can't do alone, or he goes into a home, and we don't want those things, do we?'

She nods. Again I say the most reassuring thing I can think of. The sad, true thing I say to myself when the next step seems unconscionable. The thing I've been saying for over a year.

'It won't be for long.'

Then I cook breakfast. Mum finds a note to her from my wife in a library book she is returning; she had been using it as a bookmark. Although we are divorcing she starts reading it aloud. She isn't thinking, of course, and I am working hard to stop being so angry, so while I wish she wouldn't do this, I say nothing, and instead move across the kitchen so at least this sermon from the past is not delivered directly to my ear.

Mum follows me. I focus on the vegetarian sausages as she keeps reading the letter, a note of benign content, if not aimed at me –

'I hope you are well . . . lots of love . . .'

Still, it's triggering. Regret rises so readily of its own accord that I overreact to any outside stimulus of it.

Mum shuffles closer, intoning like some crazed nun, the note an article of faith. The arrangement of the kitchen is such that I am cornered, and as I am thinking I will have to say something and what I say will not be right, she sighs and says, 'Anyway . . .', rips the note apart and tosses it in the bin. It was that she was closing in on. Not me. She would have done all this even if I was not here.

A lesson, then. But also a reminder. She has always ripped things up before she throws them away. This used to distress me as a kid. Drawings, comics, anything which she deemed worthless and in which I had invested some totemic power, shredded and gone. I wonder if it means something to her, the auto-tearing, as the pedal bin closes over the shreds. An acknowledgement that there is no going back, and so a means to move on.

5 October 2018

In the days leading up to Dad's release it becomes clear to me that for all I want to leave I have invested so much of myself in the situation that it is becoming hard to let go. I write emails with ideas about how best to care for him that feel like letters of resignation. Unlike the failed famous, I would be leaving to spend less time with my family. I identify now as the person who does 'all this', and I can feel the resistance in me to hearing my siblings out, or to handing things over and letting Mum figure matters out for herself. All of which is at best unwise and probably unfair. It is also, in practice, delusional.

This is not something that can be won, or fixed, only ridden and respected as best one can. After a while here it becomes like trying to reason with a wasp or write rules for liquid. However noble your intentions, there is an aspect that you cannot reckon. Your so-called soul becomes a spectacle, yelling at the ocean like King Canute (who at least set out to prove his limitations). You must give a little and let go a lot. There is a strange, slim line between tyranny and good intentions, between action and acting out. What we think of as passion is often just pathology.

Perhaps I cannot step firmly into the future because I am holding on to all of this.

Considering that, I chance across an essay by Toni Morrison in which she writes of earning money for her family while she was still a child. 'The pleasure of being necessary to my parents was profound,' she recalls. 'I was not like the children in folk-tales: burdensome mouths to feed, nuisances to be corrected, problems so severe that they were abandoned to the forest. I had a status that doing routine chores in my house did not provide – and it earned me a slow smile, an approving nod from an adult. Confirmations that I was adultlike, not childlike.'

She and I could, in some respects, scarcely be more different. Yet, as her references reflect, the process is primal, universally so. The will to power within one's family, the fear that every child knows of being lost or left behind, is set to rest through a sense of having value. There is nothing geographical to that one. Nor does it get old. What's odd, or just more common than we realize, is that this still holds true in middle age. It is the kid in me, perhaps, who thinks he needs to be here to be needed. The adult, such as he is, might do well to walk away.

We do our best to cope with the mortality of those closest to us from the moment it strikes us they'll die. We are used to that, one way or another. The question as we care for our elders (since we can't allow ourselves to feel too clearly ahead of time the full pain of their departure) is less *that* they die, but how. And if we are beside them for as long as that takes, our lives are bound into that bargain.

To come home and care and think that everything that was or is beneath that roof is now your problem is the high road to one's own health collapsing. It is good to do what you can, but this can only be accomplished by what one also lets go. Since I can, I must get out.

If I'm leaving I will leave thoroughly and make sure everything possible is in place. This foot regimen is complex. For clarity and unity I buy a printer to spell things out. I am shocked to discover one can be had for twenty-seven pounds. I'm aware they get you later with the ink costs, but as ever I am hedging here that none of this has far to run. I am not paying for it anyway. Mum hands me the cash and waits behind Rymans, eyes peeled and engine on.

'There were some odd-looking people hanging about,' she says when I return to the car. 'So I pretended to be reading the logbook.'

★

I rattle off copies for Mum and Dad to study the new vascular values and the way things must be. I leave another copy for the carers and email everyone else in the equation. In one of those grand gestures which work very well at times, my brother buys Dad a riser/recliner armchair that has switches and gears and plugs into the mains and that will guide him down from and lift him up onto his frame. With an hour's visit from the carers every morning and three more half-hourly calls throughout the day for food, meds and the toilet, this, we can but hope, will be OK.

In the end I am offered another fortnight's work, so the deal is sealed, the decision out of my hands. I don't just want to but now must be away when he returns. The stage is set for the last act, if that is what is coming. Iron thrones and kind hands until the final, calorific curtain. The big-biscuit goodbye. It is perhaps the last right worth having, the right to give up on life and pass on in your own fashion. And yet, even that might still depend on what it does to those around you. How long is too long when the manner of one's death is embedded in the quality of another's life?

'In the Event of Deterioration'

21 October 2018

Dad comes back. I come back too. Things, while functional, are far from happy. Mum frets over the care schedule as if she is running a small airport, scrutinizing the names and times of each arrival with a magnifying glass instead of relaxing and letting things be, as we had hoped. The house is her domain. If it happens here, she wants to know about it. Some old habits die hard, others not at all. She'll say, 'One o'clock, Tanya,' to herself. Then forget and go back: 'One o'clock, Tanya,' again, and again.

Dad sleeps or stares at the floor. He will ascend from the automatic armchair and shuffle to the toilet with help as the rota dictates, but that's about it. They are reverting to type. Something and nothing, the unstoppable and the immovable. Juxtaposed to the end.

He eats cereal and fruit and prescribed protein shakes to make up the nutritional numbers. 'High energy drinks,' Mum calls them, which conjures visions of the up-tempo gay scene of early eighties New York – a reality so distant from our own that I am reduced to inner giggling when she uses this term, which, like all else spoken here, is repeated many times a day.

No such laughs for the Old Man. His disenchantment is profound. All mirth migrated. Those calories, by any means necessary, he scarcely wants at all.

'He won't even look at bacon now,' says Mum.

Any suggestions to try this, or that, or go somewhere, are met with glum refusal.

'I could drive you to the sea?' suggests my brother.

'I've looked at the sea my whole fuckin' life.'

Mum takes charge of the remote control and he sits silently or sleeps while she watches what she wants. I ask him how he is this morning. He starts crying and says –

'I want to die.'

I don't know what to do about that. Positive words come from my mouth, but I don't know who they're for or if I mean them. There is something in his look that says, 'You would cry too if this happened to you.' I do not doubt it. Equally I am determined that I, and future me, will not resemble this. Life has dealt with much of that already. There will be no troubled sons or daughters by my side when the time comes.

This is perhaps mine and my father's saddest commonality. My wife and I lost kids in early pregnancies, he had a mother he never knew. They weigh heavily, these absent unknowns. God forbid we should discuss that.

'Chin up,' I say, and head to the kitchen.

'Door!' he says, which means close the door, please, I am in a draught.

He cannot stand to have the door open any more than Mum or I can remember to close it every time, so this is now our most persistent riff. He may not want to be alive, but he has very fixed ideas about how things should be while he is with us.

'Door . . . door . . . biscuit . . . door!'

I stick another wriggling resentment in the sack, which writhes with stifled curses and flicked Vs like a bag of cats for drowning.

22 October 2018

The hospital consultant visits Dad at home, which, if we are now to host the work that previously fell to them, is bitter-sweet. Nice to have an expert in the house, if not for this reason. I'm not there when it happens but he writes extensive notes about how things might go down.

'In the event of deterioration, he [Dad] does not want to be admitted to hospital even in the case he may die. Therefore I would advise referral to Urgent Response at the time to clinically monitor and support probable increased care needs.'

Mum is miffed by this, which may well be the understatement of this waning year since Dad doesn't discuss any of it with her. The doctor's visit is the first she knows of the 'Advanced Care Plan'. I try to figure out what dying at home might mean.

23 October 2018

There is a district nurse who knows Dad well; she and I discuss his options. Given that his most frequent problem is his circulation, how does not treating that and the open wounds that follow from its failure pan out?

'Sepsis and death,' she says, not uncheerfully. I think I saw them play live.

'How long will that take?'

'Weeks, months,' she shrugs. 'But you would be fully supported.'

No doubt. I wonder if this is really what he has in mind when he says he wants to die. This creeping, rotting end is some distance from the cut-and-dried drama of the DNR. It sounds awful. For him. For everyone who would be around it.

I try to talk to Mum about it over lunch.

'What do you think we should do about looking after Dad?'

'Well,' she says, as she zeroes in on the fruit bowl. 'He just has a banana now.'

In a blessed turn of events one of the carers, a woman who lives nearby, has taken up much of the increased rota and, as well as having a certain whispering way to get the Old Man onside, is quickly becoming a bona fide friend to our mother. They have fun. At times I hear them laughing downstairs and I'm jealous.

I recall how a friend who nursed her father said to me when this began, 'You'll learn a lot about yourself.' And how. As the layers of self recede, we are full of surprises. The last eighteen months have felt like personal archaeology at gunpoint. It is high time to put Humpty back together and get out of here again.

I take the Super Carer (and she is indisputably that) aside

and ask how this kind of slow death deal goes down. What happens when he is too weak to stand with assistance?

'Then it needs two of us,' she says. 'Some people build a hoist.'

So that would be eight people a day, at least, and structural work. More care home than family home, and thus I think a case for the latter. I file (bin) that thought like I do all ideas about the long-term future and get out for the evening to a house where there are young people.

Fearful Odds

Dave is just three months younger than me, but that counts. As do his kids, out for the night and asleep upstairs but as felt in his house as old age is in ours. I sink into his sofa, drink, and watch whatever he is watching on TV.

Tom Cruise is saving the world again. Something he says seems especially prescient.

'Everybody dies,' he exclaims, pointing to an inhuman, alien presence. 'The thing is to die well.'

Morgan Freeman emerges, much to the alien's dismay, and a huge bomb is triggered, at which point the movie, as is often the case in science fiction, reaches back into antiquity to make its point.

'How can man die better,' asks Tom as he surrenders his life, 'than facing fearful odds, for the ashes of his fathers and the temples of his gods?'

I recognize these lines. I check online. They are from Thomas Babington Macaulay's 1842 poem, *The Lays of Ancient Rome*, and concern Horatius' and his fellow Romans' defence of a bridge in 509 BC. Horatius survived the battle, but Macaulay's words have long been deployed to inspire those facing things they almost certainly will not. Unsurprisingly, my thoughts turn to my father.

How Can Man Die Better? happens to be the title of one of his favourite books, an account of the Zulu Wars. It sat in the pile beside his chair until my sister tidied it away. This was all it took for Dad to forget that he had read it, order another and read it all over again. That second copy sits beside him still, but I had never seen this coincidence of title and reality quite so clearly as I do now on another sofa, across town.

This then, is how things really end. Not like the movies Dad and I have watched together and apart in that front room. No heroics, no cavalry, bar-room brawls or military missions. Instead, a progressive decline. A cell at a time. No stirring soundtracks but a long march of indignities scored by a rising, pointless pain. You dream of saving your unit, or your planet, or going down with your ship, but instead we steer you to the toilet and it's a wonder if you make it. How can man die better? Any way but this.

I cycle back, full of wine and abstract vengeance and nothing to do with any of it but carry on.

5 November 2018

Now Dad can't open a letter we, the kids, must do the admin. I have changed the broadband deal so that I can stare into the Internet abyss for as long as I want, but my sister spots that the bills are still excessive. I dig into the numbers and deduce that part of this is from a smartphone Dad bought last year but couldn't master. He is still paying for it.

I call the phone company. My previous conflicts with them, before the fall, seem as tinted and far gone as any childhood summer, although just months ago. The person on the phone says there is a charge for ending the contract.

'He's really ill,' I say.

'How ill?' they ask.

'Terminally.'

Which is true, in its way, but the first time I have said it. The phone company waive the charge. But the sound of myself announcing the end of my father to save thirty pounds a month has, like the phone call in the supermarket, caught me off guard and is all the harder for it.

I sit upstairs where he will never come again and grind through the gears of grief. My bedroom faces west, and I have watched many a sunset through the trees from here, always more vivid when scattered through the barren boughs of winter. I slip myself into neutral and then it hits me.

We might share a stage, me and the Old Man, but he, or something in him, is directing his film, while I am making mine. We might not be in any recognizable genre but this is our drama and our hour. These rooms and chairs and old, recurring suburb views become Rourke's Drift and D-Day too. Wherever life takes you, it is your watch, your submarine movie, your Elsinore, Wembley and Waterloo.

'These people aren't heroes,' my sister likes to remind me when she reads about the worst things the best-paid football players do.

'We all are,' is my stock reply, and this is one of those occasions when I hold this to be true.

Fearful Odds

Then I understand that the man who must die better here is not him, but this quailing, questioning, vengeful incarnation of myself. When you are unambiguously reminded that the world and those with whom we share it are, as ever, out of our control, all that's left to steer, and all there ever was to change, is you.

Sad Tale's Best for Winter

'I've figured it all out!' I tell my therapist. She looks at me patiently and says –

'Don't underestimate this, the death of your father. Don't hide from legitimate feelings or pretend that sadness isn't "you".'

As ever, she is on the money, and I find myself subject that same evening in London to what might mildly be called the blues. The difference between tonight and every other troubled night is that now, for the first time, I don't see it as coming from outside me. For I don't know how long I have framed this feeling as a visitor: hostile, powerful and poised like a bandit to steal anything good that I have farmed. But this is not some scowling stranger in a black hat and outrageous spurs. It is me. And if it is me, then it is mine to fix; then one day, soon, there will be something I can do.

My sister holds the fort. She emails and calls, says it is 'chaos'. Sometimes all she needs to cope is just to talk about it this way.

Sad Tale's Best for Winter

2 December 2018

The Old Man's bowels have reasserted themselves as the prime source of devilment. Despite the schedule of care, things explode when there is no one there. So he sits or lies amid the indignity. Or worse, Mum gets involved and does the best that she can. I catch this full on, several times. Oddly, or perhaps not, there is something so inarguably grounding about cleaning up shit, that I no longer think of it as the worst of things we have to do. We even have a laugh.

'How's everything else?' I like to ask in the midst of each hygienic restoration.

I'm tidying him up this morning, proud of myself, when his colon, as if conscious of my deadly sin, launches a belated, sudden second front which catches me in the face.

'My nose is running,' says Dad, naked, spread up against the tiny toilet wall like a suspect.

I tell him his nose will have to wait a minute, and wipe mine clean.

There might be a better way, though, and that torments me. To see the need for change is one thing, to feel the pain of it is quite another. The laundry alone this present predicament generates consumes a ton of time and energy. Sheets and clothes hang from everywhere things can hang from. The mess spreads into carpets and across floors. The house is hot and damp and smells outrageous sometimes. Mum fighting this, at ninety, stooped, in rubber gloves, is a sight I too often come home to.

The Super Carer and her colleagues definitely see their share of action. I think Dad prefers that we, his family, are spared it too. It bears remembering that whatever blame and nuance might be bound up in the situation, this is not what anyone set out to do.

3 December 2018

The Old Man resists all overtures to eat something other than biscuits, protein shakes, bananas and porridge. I cook sizzling meals in an effort to clear the air and lure him back to real food. Nothing doing. The clack of his frame on the tiled floor as he is marched to the toilet rings with portent like a military drum. I am not convinced this is the right way to live. I am not convinced by this Advanced Care Plan business either. I want a clearer sense of what to do if this gets worse and even if it gets no better.

I talk on the phone with a friend who, along with his Dad, cares for his Mum. His father has gone on holiday for some respite. I ask where to.

'Auschwitz.'

He isn't joking, but we do laugh.

'He always wanted to go.'

Even so.

I find myself looking at biscuits, wondering if there is one that can expedite a blissful, sweet and overwhelming conclusion. Some days I feel my father is like some collapsing star, an astronomical phenomenon, pulling us all towards him.

'You hand him a lot of power,' notes my therapist.

Easy for her to say, but not untrue.

Sad Tale's Best for Winter

4 December 2018

Mum and I are sitting in the kitchen. Her hearing is on form and we have a good, honest chat about there being no way to know what to do. No 'right' thing. She looks into space, down her many years, and sighs.

'I thought my dad was a pain in the arse,' she reflects, uncharacteristically. Adding, 'Family life . . .'

'It's like the Mafia,' I say. '"Just when you think you are out"' – I do the Al Pacino gesture – '"they pull you back in."' If we were gangsters, Mum, we would have killed each other by now.'

'There's light at the end of the tunnel, then?' she laughs.

'Only for Sicilians,' I say.

18 December 2018

Christmas comes, or looms, depending on your point of view. A generous friend in London who has given me his keys is in a Shakespearean stand-off with his own kids, teenagers, which is in part why he has a spare room. We exchange a lot of texts about our respective and sometimes intersecting dilemmas. On one occasion I find myself wondering to him what family, in the end, is really for.

'Is it,' I ask, in the vernacular of governmental failure, 'fit for purpose any more?'

I think on this after I have sent it. The answer, of course, is of course. But it depends on what we hold to be the purpose of it all.

A value of family life might be that it holds our feet to the fire, the kind of fire we might otherwise put out or run away from, which can be just the kind we need. The acts of kindness or forgiveness needed to stick by or even mentally detach from those with whom we are principally engaged, are the stem cells of transformation. Maybe. Equally, I know there are families that should be escaped. Ours I don't think is among them. At least, not yet.

Back in the brick-built womb, I have been slowly and painfully reborn, kicking and screaming all the way. Nor, for any of this insight, does the process appear to be over. I might have cut the cord at last. And now I must grow up. Once I accept this, like the first pillar of recovery, stranger truths come.

'They're making a musical of *Only Fools and Horses*,' Mum tells me. Three times in a row.

20 December 2018

I'm having tea with Helen – the doctor, she has months left to live now – and another friend of hers. We talk about the endgame. Her friend says his parents lived in Europe.

'They told us they were going to kill themselves when they got old.'

'Did they mean it?' I ask.

'Me and my sister asked them not to. We thought they'd abandoned the idea. And then, one day, having organized their affairs, they did it just the same. We found them both neatly dead together, along with a list of instructions.'

For a microsecond, I think I might be jealous, and then the truth of this comes.

'They robbed me of the chance to care for them,' he says, clearly hurt and unhealed.

I go home more certain than ever – this cannot be won, only participated in. Every yesterday must be demolished, and each clean, forgiven day begun again. The sheets and the shit are nothing compared to the emotional laundry.

What then do we talk about when we talk about love? Beyond the poets and the propaganda and into the piss and practicalities of life. We toss the word around as if we owe it something and find ourselves wanting on the quiet. We need a better definition, or maybe none at all. Something that includes the human obstacles to clear feeling. A love that leaves us free to act, an act that frees us from the shame of falling short again.

With this in mind I come to a decision. Mum's exhaustion, the muddle of how to manage these last days, it seems naive and avoidant not to discuss residential care. If only as a respite option. I think on Dad's old wisdom, 'sometimes there's nothing you can do'. There is a flipside to that, of course.

Sometimes you can.

Mission Statement

27 December 2018

I've written a letter over Christmas. I share copies with everyone: brother, sister, Mum and Dad. The written word sidesteps the deafness and the physical and emotional logistics of getting all of us in a room.

. . . there are very real limits to what can be done here to accommodate increased needs on Dad's behalf and ensure a viable environment for Mum at the same time. We must face up honestly and unsentimentally to the fact that while the both of you being alive and well is a great blessing, your very different and sometimes antagonistic needs now mean that a time may come when this is not sustainable under the same roof, and may even be dangerous, irresponsible and counterproductive.

That said, there are things which can happen which might forestall the need for such a difficult decision, and options which mean that those decisions might not be so difficult after all. Let's remember there was a time when carers visiting seemed challenging, but in the end, that has worked out well.

One future option is for a carer to come and live at the house, there is room upstairs, and this need not be as intrusive as one might imagine if we can find the right person – and obviously we would do so. Certainly, it would remove a level of concern and danger (for us children, at least) about what can happen when the carers are not around at present or I'm not here, both for you, Dad, and for Mum.

That said, there may come a time – as outlined above – when one person is not enough to do what's needed, so then it might be a case of someone living here and carers visiting as well for lifting and so on. The question for you both is how much of that can you (especially Mum) realistically put up with? At what point is there a compelling argument for residential care, and what exactly does that mean? There are bigger and more connected outcomes here for all of us, than what any one of us, at a particular moment, might feel they want . . .

I cannot, I feel, say fairer than that, and cannot in good conscience say less. I suggest we take a day or so to absorb and reread, and then have a discussion. Meantime I go to Chris's. Again I am confronted by Tom Cruise, now in his latest impossible mission. Not for the first time in the franchise the team use 3D projection tech to convince a villain they are somewhere they are not. If it were real, this might be perfect for the elderly. If you barely interact with your surroundings yet they have become important to you, might not imitation be the most efficient form of flattery? You could be in a clean, generic, professional facility that looks just like your cluttered front room, and never know the difference.

28 December 2018

'Some birds hop,' says Mum, surveying the daily fracas around the coconut half that dangles by the drive, 'some birds walk, like this one,' she frowns at a starling, 'a bit cocky. I like the ones that hop.'

I steer her from ornithological judgement to the front room where Dad has been cleaned, fed and placed, as ever, in position.

'He just has a banana for lunch now,' says Mum.

'I know.'

We sit where we have sat for years, but today have new material, fresh terrain to hoe.

'It makes sense,' says Dad, sadly, of the letter. I can hardly believe what I'm hearing.

'We don't want someone else living here,' they say together.

'I would be thinking about them all the time,' says Mum. 'What are they doing? Have they eaten?'

'So what about the residential option?'

Dad says quietly, 'I could go and see.'

I had been expecting one of the hardest, most painful conversations of our lives, but instead comes this agreement. He will take one for the team, for Mum. Maybe even for me. I am suffused with relief, love (or what purports to be love but might just be getting what you want) and, God help me, triumph. I, the youngest, have done the impossible, grown-up thing. I can already picture myself telling other troubled children how I figured all this out. A possible TV series, like those people who can make toddlers behave.

My sister has appraised the local homes and found a nice one that is hard to get into. You must apply in advance, even for respite, like some sought-after public school. I hand him its radiant brochure, which makes the place look like a destination rather than some detention centre. So this is it. Game almost over. Good for me. Good for us.

I feel invincible. So much so, I try and fix the shower, which comes free of its moorings and strikes Mum on the head sometimes. I get the old unit off, go to the DIY store, get another and am in the early stages of installing it when something goes wrong and I realize I have no idea what I am doing. I call John. He comes around and has it up in minutes. Mum is delighted. I am delighted. There is nothing we cannot do.

I am upstairs writing in the small bedroom, all these disparate notes and confessions seeming now to coalesce toward some useful sense, a story even, when Mum shuffles in.

'I want to give you something.'

Please not money, I think, not now, after what I've done. Instead she comes back with a bag of cough sweets the carer once recommended to her and which Mum heartily endorses. I've heard all this before.

'Keep them with you,' she says, like someone handing you a magic artefact in a film. 'You look tired.'

She comes towards me and gives me a hug. I haven't slept in this room for nearly forty years, but it dissolves, this interval. I may as well be seven again. I hope it's good for her too. Still being Mum.

The previous night she had looked at my clothes and then warned me about the weather.

'It gets cold, you know.'

'I'm familiar with the climate, Mum.'

Ten minutes later I was out on my bike, freezing.

29 December 2018

Maybe this is it. An act break, in movie terms. No longer can the anti-hero hide from himself, and having found his courage and healed the present he turns to face a future he could never have imagined.

I am feeling pleased with myself when the Super Carer, on her lunchtime visit, gives me a conspiratorial nod in the hall.

'Your dad's not happy,' she says. 'He says you're putting him in a home.'

Not true.

'I know that,' she says. 'But he's got this idea.'

'Leave this with me,' I say, and walk confidently to the living room.

'I am not going anywhere,' he announces.

This comes with an outbreak of eye contact, so I know he is deadly serious.

'This is my home. I want to die here.'

'But you're not dying, are you?' I counter. 'And we were only talking about a week.'

'I don't care,' he says. 'I'm not going.'

I'm proud to see him so decisive, but not at the expense of what seems to be a healthy scheme. Is this the stand I have long wished to see him taking? Just not against me. I know deep down the illusion of a clear, clean future is dissolving, but it hasn't sunk in yet. I feel no rage or pain, but I am certain they are saddling up. I go on calmly.

'You told the carers I was making you do this?' I am embarrassed by this more than annoyed.

'You can't make me do anything,' he says.

'I have power of attorney.'

'Not till I'm dead,' he counters.

'That's not how that works,' I say. He launches a second front.

'Mum doesn't mind me being here.'

'That's not what she told me.'

'We discussed it,' he says.

'When?' I ask.

Then I think, never mind that, let's get her in here. I ask Mum to come in from the kitchen where she is in conference with the Super Carer who has kindly stuck around.

'YOU SAID YOU DIDN'T MIND!' says Dad for the second or third time as she tweaks her hearing aids.

This is a turnaround. While seemingly staring at the carpet he has organized a substantial web of counter-propaganda; I suddenly feel like I am fighting Vladimir Putin.

'I didn't know what you were saying,' Mum says to Dad eventually.

Then it comes, a wave of sadness as I realize what this really means. I say it as soon as I think it.

'You don't trust me, do you? After all we've been through. I won't let anything bad happen.'

He says nothing.

'If you get sicker, what are we supposed to do?'

'More carers!' he says, firmly.

'No matter what?' I look at Mum and ask her what she thinks.

'You're bullying her,' he says.

That does it. The horsemen of my inner apocalypse come at a gallop. I shut the whole operation of my being down lest the neighbourhood be torn asunder by some profane and primal scream.

There is one instinct left, the age-old urge to say something clever, and I am duly handed the perfect, resonant soap opera line:

'All my life I wanted you to come home, and now I need you to move, you won't go anywhere.'

If my recent past, and the rise of social media, have taught me anything, it is that the ability to conjure up things that sound smart is no reason to actually say them. I have, I hope, enough entry-level self-awareness not to do too much violence to our present in pursuit of a better past. Whatever I didn't get is long gone. And so this retort stays inside.

I won't, though. For the first time in my life I feel like I can't be here any more. Mum is ever sensitive to my distress. She knows far better than me that ours aren't roles you can just slip in and out of.

'What will you do?' she asks me in the kitchen.

I point towards the living room, still not entirely free from the urge to melodrama –

'I will not end up like that.'

I call a cab, say goodbye politely. Head for the train with half a mind to rob or jump beneath it. Anything not to feel like this again.

Beyond Freud and Larkin

Life gets easier when you don't expect to feel good about yourself any more. Beyond the conceit of happiness, suddenly you have free rein. For all my talk of acceptance and inner change, what comes instead is familiar, stagnant sensations in my stomach and brain. The depleted uranium of regret and rage. It is infantile stuff, that which rises when things don't go our way. Changing myself feels like dismantling the pyramids with a penknife, while anger calls like a case of dynamite. For now, I whittle on.

On the train I hammer out an email to my siblings. It emerges surprisingly calm. Key phrases include: 'I left on polite terms but my feelings were otherwise,' and, 'I'm sure it will work out.' If I can spin like this I should be in government. I am reminded of how writing brings order to inner ferment and can even take the worst of it away. Having led the Oedipal charge to incarcerate our father, I resolve to dismount and let this old year slip away.

10 January 2019

As is often the way in families, none of this gets openly discussed again. In part because things take a miraculous upswing in the weeks that follow.

Dad's bowels relent. Duly emboldened, the man himself decides he wants a haircut. A sign and signifier of self-respect, as well as that rarest of things – a voluntary excursion to the outside world.

My brother handles this. Mum goes too. It rains, and he sends me a picture of our parents sheltering in a doorway. It is, I think, the only time I have ever seen them holding hands. Looking at this sixty-year alliance, I am suddenly moved again. They might not do as I wish, but I know I can't do what they have done.

Human beings are a mystery. The more I throw what I deem to be logic at any of this, the less it seems to help. Again, one can contribute but not control. Still I step back. For almost a month I stay away. The longest time in the two years since I came back.

27 January 2019

Though I am welcome elsewhere, the house I grew up in is the only place left I feel I belong. Now at least I can choose to come here, since some of the self-doubt about why I do so has gone. 'Better one volunteer', and all that.

Much as I feel we are not facing up to certain issues, the unconditional welcome I receive makes me think some things might be better unsaid. 'So far so good,' as one says when falling from a tall building, in defiance of the looming ground. Home again, home again, jiggety jig.

Dad has gained weight, is eating better. The Super Carer says he is arguing more, and insists this is a good thing. Mum is cheerful. Things are working, then. This will be as good as it gets. It is not broken; I need not fix it. Cliché follows cliché until the outside world intervenes.

The care company, who are affordable, efficient and deliver a steady stream of kind and sometimes saintly people to help us, is taken over by another, larger company. There is nothing we can do about this. It simply happens.

We get a letter which promises nothing will change, but things immediately do. The first 'efficiency' to which we are subjected is that the printed rota of who comes when, which my mother studies like a sacred text, will no longer be posted to us. They will only email it.

I email them. They must know many of their clients are too old or infirm to have email? They ignore that, so I phone. I speak to someone who used to sound happy. Now they sound confused and depressed.

Can we pay a small amount to have a printed rota, like a bank statement?

No one knows.

I can print stuff if I'm there; my sister can, but all this leaves a bad taste. If saving the price of a stamp – itself symbolic of the age of the people your business serves– if this is your first priority, what other false and forced economies will follow?

30 January 2019

Helen, my friend, the dying doctor, to whom I had recommended the company, calls me after the takeover.

'Disaster,' she says.

She outlines the strain of the new company's regime on the woman providing most of her care, a young mother whose husband is off injured from his own zero sick pay, zero-hours job. The woman lives on the other side of the city, her travelling time isn't paid for and she is frequently diverted by having to cover other carers' missed calls.

When the new agency say they can't give Helen what she wants (and which was previously deliverable), she sacks them, contacts the carer herself, hires her privately and pays her more in cash than she was getting from the agency. This solves Helen's problem but places the rest of what now feels like a system being stifled by the quest for profit – or, if you prefer, efficiency – under even more strain.

Never and Again

The volume of Dad's care perhaps makes him less vulnerable to these kinds of tremors, I tell myself. But I am wrong. One of the good carers quits under the new regime and the whole system buckles. Carers don't come, or come hours early and insist on putting him to bed in daylight, or late and so he is left lying in his own waste. My sister is more upset about this than our parents who can, occasionally, ascend to a level of stoicism more commonly associated with saints.

'I promised him this would never happen,' she says.

Promises, I think, are sometimes just wishes made out loud. And this is not wish-fulfilment territory. This is the land of do the best you can and pray to learn from your mistakes.

The sadness of it is that the people who do come are amazing. The mayhem is a top-down issue which in an attempt to save money consigns the people it purports to serve back into the hands of fate. I put this to the staff in the office to whom we complain.

One of them is decent and committed enough that he even comes out and makes calls himself, but despite this he seems and says he is powerless to make any kind of useful change.

None of the carers gets a coherent schedule any more than we do now, and they are all expected, and it seems contractually terrorized, to cover for systemic mistakes. Looking after old people feels sometimes like running a failing business; it is only ever going one way. When the business you turn to for help with that is failing as well, it becomes a lot to take. That the infantry of this make do on just over eight pounds an hour is astonishing. I pay a pound a minute to explain all this to my therapist then go back to haranguing the company.

Since the Old Man is still self-funding we could find another firm. In the end it is the threat of this that seems to cause enough improvement in the service for the crisis, or at least our part of it, to abate. The state-funded must simply suffer it. And even we are bluffing. We stick with it primarily because the Super Carer is so remarkable and so good for Mum. I ask her on the drive one day if she would leave the company. She says she wouldn't, but adds –

'I would hate to lose your mum.'

I know the feeling.

Between the still unmentionable residential options and the always rebuffed suggestion of someone residing with them, this will be the terrain. It could be worse, of course. This we know since we have been there, and may well be again.

6 March 2019

'I'm dizzy,' says Mum this morning on the landing, almost falling as she does so.

I see her swaying and the whole axis of life and possibility tilts with her. What would we do if she fell now? I catch her. Try and persuade her to lie down.

'No, I have to do something,' she insists.

Next she is downstairs fetching Dad a tea. I take it to him and open the window in his room. He calls me back a minute later.

'There's a fly in here,' he informs me. I say I opened the window because the room smelled. He shrugs this off.

'I'm cold.'

7 March 2019

I am awoken from a dream in which I let a criminal gang organize Dad's care, by the sound of him calling out. I run downstairs, half-naked and still in the dream, which as I wake up more I realize intersected with another one in which he was leader of some ancient clan. He had gained a lot of weight, lived in a hut and wore a big medallion. In real life things are unchanged.

'There's someone at the door,' he says.

I check. There isn't.

'You're dreaming,' I tell him. He seems annoyed with himself. I say it's fine, better to call out than not. I note there are broken biscuits in his bedding and old meds in his pill tray. Could the carers be slipping? Then two come in at the door. They had knocked and then been to the key safe. He was right. The dreams are all mine.

What is my unconscious saying? I know well enough; I can't

look grief in the eye. I am drawn instead to powerful men in fiction. I was inordinately upset when James Gandolfini died. We dump the unspeakable intimacy on strangers. For some it was Princess Diana, for me it was Tony Soprano. One person's princess is another's wise guy.

Taking Back Control

22 April 2019

My sister's increasing oversight of the situation reveals an irony which I am not unaware of in myself – the things she worries most about and reports in Mum are attributes they share. It's the same with me and Dad and so my mission is twofold: love him/do not become him. The tail end of my own marriage was characterized and accelerated by certain comparisons in this respect which could neither be unsaid nor wholly disregarded. Cleaning up your parents can be like polishing a mirror.

'Mum obsesses about the schedule,' my sister tells me, obsessively.

I have also known my sister to complain about Mum doing too much while simultaneously insisting on cooking us a meal with a broken wrist and plastered hand and then washing up afterwards, wilfully indifferent to my own chorus of 'can I do anything to help?' As ever, the main thing she needs me to do is listen.

Over a two-day period in London I am subjected to a stream of metadata in respect of Dad's indignant bowel, updates which are also going back and forth between the care company, the

Super Carer, the GP, district nurses, and our brother. When there is eventually movement, so many people are aware of this – the shit heard around the world – that there is a palpable mood swing across much of southern England. I have seen less detailed reporting of royal births.

When I get back, the household's glare has shifted from the toilet to the television. After months of disinterest Dad suddenly asks for the TV remote control and a refresher course in how to use it.

It was glued to his palm once. To see him lose all sense of how it worked was troubling; his interest in using it again is encouraging. Less so perhaps for Mum, who has enjoyed the relative calm and televisual autonomy his apparent decline had enabled. Suddenly he's keen again. Let's not get in the way of that. Even if it might mean watching *High Noon* first thing in the morning for the rest of our lives.

An inspection of the remote reveals buttons worn blank and down to nubs from his relentless pressing (Mum favours the traditional channels and so has no use for the more elaborate control). Dad is not only back, he wants full digital dominion.

I try to use it, but it won't work, except by applying the kind of pressure with your thumb that could shatter a walnut. I order a new one. Amazon, somehow still thriving despite Dad's withdrawal, gets it here in hours. I try to walk him through it.

'This button means pause . . .'

'I have no memory,' he announces, matter-of-factly.

'OK, this button—'

'Could you write it down?'

I count calmly through my frustration. I was momentarily pleased with myself for getting a new remote, 'stunning high definition back at your fingertips'. Now this achievement, like so many others, has vanished into the swamp of fresh (and ancient) problems. Also, I am supposed to be going out.

I print out a picture of the remote and draw lines connecting each button to an explanation of its function. Whilst I am at it I also cancel a diabetic eye appointment he has decided he doesn't want to go to. Blindness is now preferable to getting out of the house, it seems. You end up not questioning this stuff. No point my dying of frustration before the end of the ride. We've come too far together for that.

I hand him the paper and tell him the appointment is cancelled. He squints at the printout and the remote control.

'I can't see anything,' he says.

Maybe you should go to that eye appointment, is what I want to say, but instead we step through the workings of the remote on paper.

'Isn't there some appointment we have to cancel?' interrupts Mum.

I go to the kitchen to calm down. When I come back Dad has got the TV working. Or at least a paused image of Huw Edwards.

'Why is he on?' says Mum, annoyed. 'It isn't time for the news.'

Indeed. Dad is paused in a recording. We work through it.

'We've seen this!' says Mum.

She sneers at the screen. Despite her late-life penchant for

verbal repetition, she never did like the idea of seeing something twice. Hence her long resistance to video recorders.
While some women camped out against nuclear weapons,
video was my mother's dreaded eighties bomb. In the end,
neither campaign was successful. Now here we are in the
present, looking at the past again.

'This is an exact replica of yesterday!' she announces. Tell
me about it.

'I understand!' says Dad, stabbing all the wrong buttons,
putting aside the instructions. Grease from the latest Scottish
biscuit already leaking through the paper.

'Where are your glasses?' I ask, this seeming central to the
problem, since the new remote cannot be to blame.

'Upstairs?' he says, adding, 'I don't know.'

He hasn't been upstairs in over a year. If the glasses are
there then he doesn't need them. I have had my coat on for
so long now in anticipation of leaving, that in the heat of the
lounge I am almost fainting. Huw Edwards shimmers in the
corner like a mirage. I run outside.

It's raining. I am moving through town on my way to see
a movie, a restored Western, of all things, drinking in fresh
air and freedom, when Dad phones.

'What button do I press?'

'I can't see you and it's raining,' I explain.

'Oh,' he says, something in his tone suggesting that neither
ought to be an obstacle to his viewing.

I say we'll sort it out when I get home.

I get the control thing. With so much gone by the wayside
the tiniest dominion must be madly tempting. The world

outside indifferent, you in your chair. Your body a network of cells you don't even manage any more and few diehard, hand-picked loyalists in the cave to do your biscuit bidding.

I get back and the TV is working fine. He's cracked it.

'Can we cancel that eye appointment?' he asks for the millionth time.

As ever, the appointment I must cancel is with my own reaction. To run the world inside us, not the household, or the country. That, they say, is real control.

Sweetness Follows

6 July 2019

Somehow the centre of this sickly system holds. Weeks become months which pass with matters much the same, and this becomes all one could wish for. Things are stable, the care company recovering, and we so seasoned that in July we attempt to get Mum out of the house overnight, something that hasn't happened for two years. The occasion is my nephew's wedding. Through a deft and orchestral effort of our collective attributes and dysfunctions, this goes OK. Slow and stubborn learner that I am, I allow myself to think that this recent success means everyone is something close to happy, that things might be all right.

27 July 2019

I wake up at a friend's house in London, due to head home this afternoon since my sister is on holiday, and see my phone is full of missed calls from my mum and brother.

'Dad's taken an overdose,' says Mum's message.

She has called the paramedics. My brother's message says

that he is on his way to them. I numbly, nauseously throw on some clothes. I am two or three hours away from home. No idea what I will need for this trip at all.

I move slowly and cannot make simple decisions. Shock gives way to sadness that he might have already died or be dying right now as I am trying to remember everyday things to take with me to whatever this turns out to be. Sadness turns to an overwhelming sense of futility.

What comes next, and takes me by surprise, is admiration. I imagine what his process might have been. He must have waited until he knew I was coming because he trusted me to deal with this, to make the aftermath OK. Maybe *this* is when I finally grow up. A posthumous and profound act of parenting. I find myself hoping that it has worked, and he has died and is not instead trapped or stranded in some nether state, bound to stay there indefinitely or reawaken to a world and in a body he hoped never to see again.

My brother phones.

'Panic over,' he proclaims.

I haven't panicked so much as shut down. I take it this means Dad isn't dead. He had taken, it transpires, four temazepam. Enough for a deep doze but not for a send-off. He was awake by the time the paramedics and my brother arrived. This is officially chalked up as an accident, but –

'He told me he had chosen the coward's way out,' reports my brother.

So there was intent. I told my dad I was going to do this once, suicide, years ago. He said that was the worst day of his life, so fair's fair.

What brought this on, worse pain, fresh despondency, clear thinking?

'No,' says my brother. 'He thought you were coming back to put him in a home.'

If we weren't still talking I'd be speechless. It has been seven months since that option was stopped in its tracks, even as a discussion. How has it come to this? I know we are long past the point of expecting our parents' minds to conform to the rigours of reality. But still.

'I thought he'd timed it so I could help sort it out.'

'You thought you were the hero!' laughs my brother.

Anything but.

'Trust me, in a few days no one will even remember,' he says.

I will. As memories dissolve around me, there's a lot I can't forget. I want to give up, withdraw, shut down. Protect myself in some way.

On the train I feel baffled, beaten. I was happier when I thought it was more serious. This is just more of the same, seemingly endless situation. The whole enterprise, thousands of hours, dozens, even hundreds of players convened over years to facilitate a solution, and in the end, the person that you think it's for concludes that you are out to get them. And I must accept that they are entitled to that. No matter what you do, in the end it's out of your hands. Do your best, calmly, I think to myself. Then surrender to the outcome.

Calm is elusive as the cab rolls past the crematorium and towards the house. Would I sooner be making the turn in a hearse? I can just about repeat the serenity prayer as I walk through the door.

Sweetness Follows

His chair is empty so he's still in bed. Again I think of *Apocalypse Now*. Martin Sheen coming upriver to Marlon Brando, at last approaching the temple where the general has made his final, feral stand. Two lines from the narration spring to mind. 'It smelled like slow death in there,' which feels right, and, 'I don't see any method at all.' And I can hear the music of the Doors that scores the film's finale and beginning. 'This is the end . . .'

Mum (filling in for Dennis Hopper in the movie analogy) intercepts me in the hall before I can see him.

'Now then, there's been a mix-up with the medicine.'

I am not sure if she is running propaganda here or has genuinely forgotten that we've spoken. It doesn't matter.

It is as if all the other repetitions and misunderstandings have built to this, a kind of event horizon in which no truth lasts longer than the instant of its utterance or any further than its perceiver. To consider that a so-called fact might matter, or endure, will only bring new pain. We are entirely of the moment now.

The old pain is still there, though, indignant and abiding. There is so much ephemera, equipment and outright crap about my father's bed that you can no longer sit beside it. I perch on its edge, which feels uncomfortable. For us both, no doubt, in every sense.

There he lies, haloed by shortbread crumbs and foil fragments from blister packs. The light, as ever, is good in here. The room we made just over a year ago looks like a modern old master. Caravaggio via the biscuit aisle. We hold hands as best he can and he gazes at me, eyes caulked with chemical sleep, and says –

'Don't put me in a home.'

So, he has placed the unknowable (death) above the imaginary (care home). The things we'll do for the ideas we've made. It's pathetic, in the sense of: 'arousing pity, especially through vulnerability or sadness'. As opposed to: 'miserably inadequate'. How those two interpretations can live within the same beholder. All the distance and proximity between love and judgement inside that single word.

My brother is right. An hour from now this is unremembered. Mum stops rattling around the house like a screen saver rebounding against the margins of a monitor, and is instead singing in the kitchen. Dad, assisted by the Super Carer, has made it to his chair, where he calls for the TV listings. Suddenly there is a future. Even if it is just tonight's television.

'Seagulls are getting more upfront,' says Mum as she rifles through the newspaper. 'One has carried a chihuahua away.' Upfront, as if this was their agenda all along, and they are just getting around to it.

I wonder if some mythic bird could come and take me or the Old Man to some other land. A good end for a sailor. Real Sinbad stuff. For now, I wipe the sleep from his eyes and tell him all I want is for him to stay.

'I am a weak character,' he apologizes, but it comes out as a statement.

'No, you're not,' I tell him.

You're strong enough. Enough to hold your own story. Enough to carry a book.

Those Lovely Wounds

Next morning's carer is an hour and a half late, not uncommon on a Sunday. Mum blames the individual; I blame the system. Business very much as usual. I'm still fizzing with the dissonance of yesterday. Looking for an argument, somewhere to dump it all. The carer arrives. No harm done.

'You never know what the day holds,' says Mum brightly when they've gone.

I realize then she is still teaching me. I talk of letting go, but here she is again, way ahead of me. Living it. I ask Dad if he is OK. He seems a little hesitant, perhaps self-conscious. Says he's fine. I go to the shop with Mum. He phones my mobile on the way.

'Liquid soap,' he says, then keeps repeating it: 'Liquid soap! LIQUID SOAP!'

As though it was running at Aintree and he wanted me to put a bet on. Liquid Soap, fiver each way. I buy some. Evidently he is OK. We are safely back to normal. Perfectly repositioned in the everyday.

Except I am not. Something still roils inside. I call a friend who has been through all this before, even the attempted parental suicide. We talk about the de-skilling. How the elderly realm is strange territory, another dimension where you can learn the language, but cannot take it with you. Something's lost as you leave. They are working with a different alphabet, a new mythology, prayer book and legal system each time you return. Each comeback feels like Gulliver's travels, except that you feel large and small in the same country. Hold to the old values, and your holding will devour you. The past, so often clung to and discussed, can drown us too.

I tell him I am writing all this down. He asks me how it ends. And it doesn't strike me till I say it:

'There is no ending.'

This isn't a myth; this is a report from the front lines. All I can say is I thought it was one way, and then it was the other.

This ungraspable business *is* the way. And we mistake that uncertainty for a disaster, for the very end of ourselves. Identities forming and dissolving like shapes in water or visions in flames. Good son, bad parent, angry brother. Nothing will ever quite fit, or last, or work for what awaits us. What is us is beyond us. Try and lay a narrative arc on that and it will finish you instead. Let it be.

I think of that advice I was given long ago – 'People don't change, they just become more of who they are.' And even this is open to interpretation. What are we in the first place, something more than dreaming meat? What is anyone becoming? Speechless dust; or earthly gods? Both at the same time?

'It doesn't end,' my friend reflects, 'even when they die.'

Those Lovely Wounds

This is a story about the dangers of story, I suggest. Where truth skins fiction's hide.

'Sounds like Beckett,' he says.

'I'll take that,' I reply.

I can't go on, I'll go on. Fail better. Into the endgame. Something far beyond gentle, into the good night.

29 July 2019

'He just has a banana at lunchtime now,' says Mum again, as if it were breaking news.

I check the calendar. Today must be the 200th time this has been so. Banana lunch bicentennial. Dad meanwhile is watching the Grand Prix so loudly it is like being at the race. Possibly louder. Mum sits and reads the paper through this somehow. I watch them and wonder what I'll do without them. Who I'll be.

We are not in the hero business here, but the less-villains game. Yet heroism surrounds us. Our mother's uneven step. Our father's broken breaths. Another fly throwing itself against the window of the living room, trying to get out. That bird still fighting its reflection, trying to get in. Life, despite everything. Then the district nurse's knock.

'That'll be the midwife,' says Dad, oblivious to his error.

The nurse rolls in, buoyant, cheerful. Operatic. Unwraps his feet and says –

'Let's have a look at those lovely wounds.'

And so I head upstairs, type this and tend to mine.

In memory of my father (1930–2021)

Follow the author @reluctantcarer and visit their website,
reluctantcarer.com.